Broken Glass

Roy Slootheer

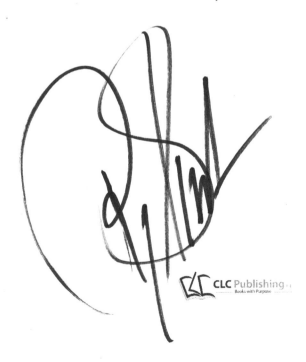

CLC Publishing
Books with Purpose

Copyright © 2020 by Roy Slootheer

All rights reserved. No part of this book may be used or reproduced in any manner whatsoever without written permission of the author.
The events portrayed within the context of this book are from the perspective of the author and depicted as his opinion only.

Published by CLC Publishing, LLC.
Mustang, OK 73064

Printed in the United States of America

Cover Design by Stellar Creative, LLC

Book Design by Shannon Whittington

ISBN: 978-1-0878-8350-2

Non-Fiction/Family and Relationships/Death, Bereavement
Non-Fiction/Motivationa/Inspirational

There's a blue rocking chair, sittin' in the sand
Weathered by the storms and well-oiled hands
It sways back and forth with the help of the winds
It seems to always be there like an old trusted friend
I've read a lot of books, wrote a few songs
Looked at my life, where it's goin', where it's gone
I've seen the world through a bus windshield
But nothing compares to the way that I see it
To the way that I see it, to the way that I see it
When I sit in that old blue chair

Kenny Chesney

For Becky

Only the few lucky ones will be blessed to enjoy the privilege to view the world through old worn windows.

Preface

We all hope, sometimes assume, that our lives will be filled with joy and that we will be blessed with good physical and mental health. That we do not run out of time before our skin becomes fragile, engraved with wrinkles of history, and our hair turns white gray. Too often we take life for granted until the sand of our hourglass unexpectedly starts to run faster. Suddenly, time is slipping away, running through our fingers rapidly. Only then, do we realize the value of time. Only then, do we discover what is truly important and what is not worth our time.

When the glass of Becky's hourglass broke, the sand of time was pouring out rapidly. Too soon, too early. This story is about her courage to face the war with cancer. About the struggles she went through while she was trying to reach for victory on the battlefield. It tells the story from my point of view, as her husband; her soulmate. Despite the fact Becky was staring death straight in the eyes, while it had its ruthless grip around her neck, choking her slowly and sucking the life out of her, she continued to be the loving and caring person she had always been. I stood by her side. Holding her hand through all the unfair bloody battles, withstanding this skin-tearing, ruthless storm, motivated by the Grim Reaper himself with his insatiable thirst for death.

I supported her with all my might. Our love only grew stronger in the midst of disaster and pain. I was blessed to have her close to my heart over the fifteen years we were together. I thank God for allowing me to be by her side, hold her hand, kiss her broken lips, and caress her fragile skin when it was time for her to travel from this world to the next.

Live your life to the fullest since no one knows when you are being called for departure.

One

My stomach was in a knot, turned upside down, as if it were rammed into a meat grinder, without regret or warning, causing an uncontrollable shiver through my body. The pounding in my chest sounded like drums pacing loudly in my ears, alarming me that my cardiac muscle was working overtime. My oxygen intake more rapid, mental focus fading, turning inward, wondering how we got here. Seconds started to feel like hours. Slowly my mind reclaimed focus, my attention aimed at him.

He stood motionless in the middle of the room, silently staring at us with an aimless, hollow gaze. As my pupils started to sharpen my vision, I noticed the uneasiness in his eyes that declared the state of emergency of the current situation. He knew how bad this was. He knew that I understood the severity of this situation from which almost no escape was possible. Only a few blessed ones were able to avoid the fatal grip of the expected end result.

Slowly I turned my head as if I were trying not to alert anyone of my movements. My attention towards her, our eyes locked, the room once again faded, sounds disappeared. Just her and I. She was thrown into this mess, unwillingly brand marked. She did not want to be here. She did not belong here. Her pupils sucked me into the depths of her soul. Although no words were spoken, their screams were gruesomely loud. A gentle squeeze from her hand into mine confirmed our connection; her trust in me and her fear for what might be coming her way. A disastrous future luring from above, like a hawk ready to dive from unknown heights to pierce his claws into his prey, from which no escape was possible; slowly and painfully ripping life from his helpless victim. Although her voice was silent, I was aware of her trembling soul inside. She placed her fears into the deep dark parts of her subconscious, unwilling to give in to the probable outcome of this horrific information.

Less than twenty-four hours ago, none of this gruesome intelligence was part of my existence. I had just started my night shift at a small local hospital where I had recently accepted a new position as an emergency department nurse. I detested the night shift, but this was just a temporary situation until I was fully trained so I could transition into my regular day-time hours. I also still worked as an ER nurse at one of the larger hospitals, but better pay and benefits caused me to change employers.

I parked my truck in the employee parking lot and walked over to the main entrance of the ER. My movement in front of the large glass doors was sensed via a motion-detector and both doors, with 'EMERGENCY DEPARTMENT' in big white letters, opened with a quick swoosh. An almost empty waiting room welcomed me. The awkward silence was eerie, almost spooky. I waved my hospital ID in front of the electronic reader on the wall. A gentle beep arose from the machine requesting a four-digit security code. As I entered the code a soft chime confirmed it was accepted. The nurses' station was straight ahead, behind glass windows, almost like a fishbowl, and conveniently located in the center of all the ER-rooms.

My backpack landed on the laminated floor with a soft thud. I placed my hands on the armrests of the chair and lowered myself into the soft leather. The computer screen stared at me, displaying a roster with all ER rooms. Only two rooms were occupied and it seemed both of them were still unassigned. My right hand controlled the mouse with small, smooth movements. Guiding the arrow on the screen onto the name in ER room 6. I assigned the patient to myself with a simple click.

On the way to meet my patient, I passed by the administrative assistant. She seemed mindlessly staring at the computer screen. I placed my hand on the counter and made a soft tapping sound with my fingers, trying to get her attention.

"I am going into room six," I said.

Without moving a muscle, she slowly lifted her eyes from the screen, almost annoyed about the disturbance of whatever she was doing.

"Okay," she confirmed and returned her focus back to the screen.

Room 6 was right around the corner from where I was standing and within seconds, I faced the light pine-colored wooden door. I wrapped my fingers around the door lever. The cold steel actually felt good as I gently pushed it down to open the door. A mild squeak from the hinges reminded me of the sound of an old musty coffin you see in vampire movies. As Count Dracula arises from his daily slumber, preparing himself for a night filled with bloodsucking of his poor helpless victims.

I stepped into the room with a delicate smirk on my face, still visualizing Dracula sitting upright in his casket with white fangs protruding from his lips. The large pine door was slowly falling shut behind me, making that same gentle squeak again. Right before it came to a complete close, I could hear a distant voice calling,

"Roy, you have a phone call on line two."

My eyes made brief contact with the young girl that was too skinny for comfort. She was wearing a blue hospital gown, covered by a blanket, holding the hand of an older gentleman whom I assumed was her father. I moved my visual contact from her to the man, then back to her.

"I am sorry," I said, "Let me get that phone call real quick and I will be right back."

The girl stared at me as if I were speaking Russian; the older man though, smiled and nodded,

"No problem."

As I turned around to leave the room, I wondered who and why someone would be calling me at work. I exited the room with a quick stride, ignoring the coffin-like squeak from the door, my eyebrows frowning, causing my forehead to have a single large wrinkle between my brows. I turned the corner heading towards the nurses' station. The receptionist clarified who was calling,

"Your friend Lisa is on line two," she said.

Although enlightened about who was calling, I was still confused about why.

With a determined step, I walked around the desk, placed my hand on the back of the closest chair, then spun it around to face me. The chair came to a sudden halt against my leg, I lowered myself into the leather seat. My hand reached out, grabbed the telephone, and placed it against my ear. I pushed the button with the red flashing light.

"Lisa, this is Roy. What's up?"

Lisa has been a close family friend for the last twelve years. When I joined the local fire department of the small town we lived in, both Lisa and her husband Matt almost instantly became friends. Most firefighters are cut from the same wood. They live for the same common goal: to help others. Frequently knee deep in blood, guts, and other body parts, but ultimately, we all have an unspoken desire to help. Yes, we like to play with fire, and yes, we are adrenaline junkies, but deep down, beyond that thick layer of coolness, we are genuine caring souls. The brotherhood and comradery amongst firefighters are tight and unique. We understand that most of us have been in a dark place where no one dares to go, but where we willingly and freely step into, just so we might be able to save another soul.

Lisa would never contact me at work unless it was really important. As she started to talk, I noticed a slight thrill in her voice. I wondered if it was from excitement or if she was nervous about something.

"Roy, I am sorry to call you at work. I tried to reach you on your cell phone several times, but I keep getting your voicemail," she explained.

"Listen," she continued, "I am really concerned about Becky."

Worried about Becky? Why? What was going on?

I leaned forward in the chair as if it would help me pay more attention to what was being said. I pressed the phone harder against my ear so I could hear better, but before I could respond, she continued,

"She has been really tired all day. It was so bad tonight that she asked me to pick up the boys to take them to dinner," she took a deep breath in and sighed with obvious anxiety, "and I know she has been sleeping on the couch all day. There is something not right, I tell you."

When I got home earlier that morning, just past 7 from my nightshift, I remember giving Becky and the boys a quick kiss before heading straight to bed. She was taking Connor and Dane to Kids

Club. I was asleep most of the day and unaware of anything that was going on.

"You know I would never call you at work if I didn't believe there was something going on with her," Lisa continued trying to make her case.

The frown on my forehead intensified, an unsettled feeling of nervousness crept into my body. That feeling you get in the pit of your stomach, as if you were about to take an important exam and you are not really sure if you are well prepared for it. My response to Lisa was fast and simple.

"Okay, I am on my way."

Without hesitation I placed the phone back onto the receiver, latched my right hand onto the top grip of my backpack, and as I stood up, swung it onto my shoulder. With a determined pace I walked towards the office of the charge nurse. As I passed the administrative assistant, I explained that I had to leave because of an emergency at home. Suddenly she became more responsive than before.

"Are you ok?" she asked with a concerned voice.

"Not sure, I hope so," I responded as I continued my resolute march to the charge nurse. Not realizing the nightmare that was waiting for me just hours away.

My shoes were making those annoying, high-pitched noises on the laminated floor. My mind did not stop wondering about what could be going on. Becky started to have an irritated dry cough just a few days ago. She went to the urgent care down the street from our house where she was diagnosed with bronchitis. As expected, she received the standard treatment of antibiotics, steroids, and some cough medicine. Four days later, there had been no improvement. Actually, the cough was getting more intense and frequent, so I told her to go back to the urgent care. After a chest X-ray was complete, they determined that she might have the beginning of pneumonia and changed her antibiotics.

I arrived at the office of the charge nurse. The door was open, papers were scattered all over her desk. On the left, attached to the corner of her desk, was a small bright yellow desk-fan. It was aimed straight at her face, causing her hair to gently move backwards in almost slow-motion flowing waves. I rapped my knuckles on the doorpost. Without any noise, she slowly turned her chair around and looked at me with a kind, gentle smile. She was an older female with white gray shoulder-long hair. Her eyes revealed the compassionate soul harboring inside. After she placed her pen down on the logbook she was writing in, she responded to my appearance,

"Hey, what's up?"

As I started to explain why I was standing there, I noticed the tremble in my speech and the slight shake in my hands; an unsolicited excitement, a feeling that I did not want, but I was sure she noticed the concern in my voice.

"Go home, take care of your wife and please let us know what is happening," she said.

I left the building through the same sliding doors as when I started my shift. I moved from the cool comfortable temperature-controlled hospital, into the sticky, humid, outside where breathing suddenly became heavier. I did not realize at that moment, when I passed through the glass sliding doors, it was going to be the last time I would walk through them as an employee.

The drive home normally takes anywhere between thirty to forty minutes, all depending on the traffic. One of the largest universities is housed here in the same town, so traffic could be thick at times. I just left the employee parking lot from the hospital, cranking my steering wheel to the right, turning onto main street, heading east towards the interstate. My brain was unable to stay still.

What's going on? What's happening?

A sudden buzz from my phone abruptly pulled me out of my trance. I reached over to grab it from the middle console. I looked at the screen, a message from Becky,

'Don't listen to Lisa. I am fine. Just really tired. Don't leave work. Love you.'

Her text made me smile, a sense of joy pushed some of the worries aside. This was so typical for her, always trying to make sure everyone is taken care of, she didn't want to be a burden to anyone. Cars in front of me came to a sudden halt. Traffic light. My opportunity to respond,

'Too late babe. I am on my way. Be home in about 30. Love you.'

Cars started to move again like a herd of cattle being pushed through metal gates, through the intersection. I placed my phone back onto the middle console, with the screen facing upward so I could keep an eye on it just in case another text message would come in. Within seconds of putting it down, it buzzed again. A quick glance to the screen and then back to focus on the road - a new message from Becky. I placed the phone in front of me, resting it on top of the middle part of my steering wheel. My eyes moved rapidly from the road to the message, quickly I read,

'Ok honey, but I really think I am fine.'

Knowing Becky, she would never ask anyone for help, but the fact that she actually agreed with me coming home was concerning. It was a clear sign that something was going on. The drive home was a long thirty minutes, no music, just silence. I didn't want to be distracted, I needed to concentrate and try to figure out what was going on.

I reached for my phone without looking and with an amazing almost robot-like precision, my hand landed on top of it. I picked it up, placed it back on the steering wheel, a single touch on the power button brought the screen to life. A picture of Becky and the boys greeted me. I smiled and felt a warm flow of joy. My lips moved and whispered,

"What is going on with you sweetie?" as if she could hear me.

I needed to call Lisa to let her know I was on my way. A simple push on the recall button and I could hear the ringtone. Lisa answered in a more anxious tone, her words rapid, as if she were out of breath.

"Are you on your way?" she asked.

"Yep. Left ten minutes ago," I responded.

"I am really sorry Roy, but I know there is something wrong with her," she said hastily.

"There is no reason to be sorry, Lisa," I explained.

I knew she only had Becky's best interest in mind.

"I will take her to the ER when I get home, but I have no clue how long it will take," I said.

"Are you okay staying with the boys tonight until we get back home?"

"I will leave right now," she said, "so I will be there before you get there."

I was planning on taking Becky to Mercy hospital in Des Moines, where I also still worked. It was much closer to us, only fifteen minutes away, and they offered a higher level of care.

The sun started to settle in the west, some small puffy clouds started to pop-up here and there, like little cotton balls stuck on a soft purple-red blanket. I slowed down right before getting to our driveway and turned onto the black asphalt, leading up to our split-level home. We had almost 5 acres just outside the city limits of the small town of Altoona, Iowa. As I pulled up to our house, I remembered that we bought this home twelve years ago. Becky was pregnant with our first son, Connor. He was planned to arrive in the second week of August in 2000. We moved into our new home in June, just in time to get the house ready for his arrival.

The headlights of my truck sliced through the darkness like a sharp blade. Lisa's red truck appeared in the light beams, parked to the right. Large concrete steps paved a curved entrance towards the front door, with bushes on both sides . I parked close to the stairs, so Becky didn't have to walk too far to get to the truck.

On any normal day, both the boys would be already in bed, sleeping and hopefully dreaming about happy things. Since it was summer break, I was positive they would still be awake running around the house with an unlimited supply of energy. I opened the front door and the faint screech released by the hinges was a signal for the boys letting them know I was home. Before my feet hit the tiles in the hallway, I could hear screams arising from the living room.

"PAPA!"

Followed by the sound of running little feet across the hardwood floor, like a herd of wild horses galloping through the pasture.

I arrived at the top of the stairs that led to the living room. I stood still as both boys charging at me. They came to a screeching halt right at my legs. Both of them were clinging to my thighs, one on each side, as if I had been gone for months. I planted a quick kiss on both of their heads.

Slowly I staggered into the living room. I was walking with both boys still attached to my legs, like two massive blocks of concrete. As I moved forward, I placed my hands on the backs of their heads, ensuring that they would not fall. Struggling to move forward in a Frankenstein-like walk, I focused my attention to my girl. She was sitting in our chair, an oversized one-seater, big enough for the both of us. Becky was sitting on her side with both her legs folded beneath her. With a big smile on her face she responded to my arrival. She was one of those few people who did not have to say anything, because her smile and eyes would light up the whole room. Anyone could feel the kindness radiating from her, like the heat from a fireplace on a cold winter's night. I moved closer to her.

"Hey babe," I said. I smiled and continued my approach to collect my kiss.

She raised both her arms up as if she were trying to attract me like a magnet. When I leaned forward, she embraced me in her arms, and right before our lips touched, she whispered,

"Hey sweetheart, thanks for coming for me."

Our lips connected, my right hand moved from holding Dane's head in one smooth motion to the right side of her face and placed it gently on her cheek.

"Are you doing ok babe? What's going on?" I asked.

Her beautiful green eyes shone like freshly polished emeralds in the bright sunlight on a crisp spring afternoon. Her joy to see me was easily detectable. I brought her comfort by coming home early that night as she knew I would take care of her. When she started to explain what was going on, I rubbed the boys' heads, asked them to let go of my legs, leaned over and planted a kiss on their cheeks. I lowered myself down onto the ottoman right in front of her.

"I don't know what is going on," she said, "I am just so tired I have a hard time doing anything. I just think it is from this stupid cough I can't get rid of. It is wearing me out."

"Well, we have to get it checked out babe," I said.

Lisa was sitting in the loveseat to the left of us. My head turned towards her, I smiled, "Thank you for coming Lisa."

"No problem," she replied, "You guys go ahead; I will stay here with the boys."

Connor and Dane always enjoyed hanging out with Lisa, she was like a grandmother to them. Almost everything was allowed and a trip to the local ice-cream store was always on the agenda. We explained to the boys why we were going to hospital; to figure out why mama was coughing so much.

"Ok, guys," I said, "we will be back in a little, but I want you both in bed around 10 tonight ok?"

Both boys looked at me and ran over to give us a big hug.

"I love you sweetie. Listen to Lisa, okay?" I said as I kissed Connor, the oldest, and squeezed him tight.

"Okay" he responded. "I love you too Papa."

He walked over to Becky. She grabbed his face with both hands, cupped around his jaw and kissed him.

"I love you sweetie. We will be back before you know it," she said, and another kiss landed on his little lips.

Dane, only 16 months younger than Connor, rested his head on my shoulder, his arms around my neck.

"I love you buddy. See you later tonight, ok?" As my lips reached his cute little face, he tightened his arms around my neck. His silence voiced his dislike of this situation.

"I love you too Papa," he whispered softly.

Becky wrapped him in her loving arms, followed by many kisses on his face.

"Love you sweetie pie. We will be back before you know it," she said.

As we descended the stairs toward the front door, I thanked Lisa again for taking care of the boys.

The air outside was still warm and humid. The sun had disappeared below the horizon, but the heat from the day was still lingering on. The stars started to appear in the east. One by one they began to light up and soon the whole sky would be wrapped in this dark blue blanket filled with shiny sparkles. We walked towards the truck with our hands interlocked. Even after thirteen years of marriage, we would always hold hands like a newly married couple.

I glanced over to my right, checking on her, making sure she was fine. Becky smiled, almost smirked, as she could feel my caring eyes gleaming all over.

"I am fine," she said without deviating her gaze forward, "don't worry."

My hand reached out for the door handle and with a persuasive and sudden jerk, I pulled the door open for my princess. While she started to make motion to step in, in the midst of her path she suddenly stopped, looked at me, placed her right hand on my cheek and smiled. Her eyes glittering, leaning forward and sealed our continuous love with another kiss. Nothing was said, but everything was understood.

Two

It was a crystal-clear night with a new moon. A shiny sliver was floating just above the horizon in the dark blue blanket. If you stared at it long enough, you would see the outline of the dark side of the moon, but in one simple glance, only the illuminated part was visible to the eye. On any given night, that would have been a cool thing to observe, but that night, I was on a mission; trying to get my girl to the ER to figure out what was going on.

The interstate turned from south bound to a westward direction. It brought you over the Des Moines river and you could see the hospital on the north side of the interstate. For years I drove this route to get to work in the ER at Mercy hospital. I never paid any attention to the structure or placement of the hospital building at all, but that night I noticed how tall and prominent it stood. The helipad on top of it was lit up like a candlestick. I knew that it meant that the helicopter was on an inbound approach.

I turned onto the road that led us to the front door of the ER. The large spotlights surrounding the hospital plastered the outside walls with bright lights, making it look like a beacon of hope in the darkened night. The parking lot was almost empty.

"Thank God honey," I said, "I don't think it is really busy tonight."

"Good," she responded, as she turned her head my way and smiled.

"I guess we will be home earlier than we thought," she continued hopefully.

I parked about 50 feet away from the ER entrance, turned off the ignition, grabbed my phone, and stepped out the truck. I walked around the front, my eyes aimed at Becky, and as I reached her side, we never lost eye contact. I opened her door and as she started to glide out from her seat, I grabbed her hand to support her.

With our hands entangled, we walked towards the entrance of the ER. Nervous but determined to figure out what was going on. Before we reached the doors, I slowed down and softly pulled back on Becky's arm, she stopped. I leaned toward her, our lips connected, then released without a sound. The glass doors opened as we got closer to the entrance. We walked through the hallway and passed the security guards' desk. It was too early for security, so it was unmanned. Normally a security guard would sit at that post in the evenings after midnight.

Only two people were in the ER waiting room. Although sitting in almost opposite corners of the waiting area, they were both staring at the same TV. This waiting room could hold up to 50+ people, and at times, during the weekend, all the seats would be filled. Every exam room would be occupied, and frequently it would be so busy that patients had to be placed in ER beds in the hallways.

As we got closer to the front desk, the triage nurse looked up. She recognized me right away and she smiled.

"Hey Roy, what are you doing here?" she asked.

I explained our reason for coming to the ER.

"Cough and increased fatigue," she confirmed while her pen was endorsing that statement on paper.

"We are pretty slow right now," she explained, "which ER doc do you want?"

At any given time, there would be about six to nine ER providers working. Divided between three ER pods, each with about ten to twelve rooms. I was pleased to see that Doctor Kawamura was working. I worked with him frequently, and besides that, he was also the medical director for the fire department.

"We will put you in room 11, the bigger one," she winked.

"Okay," I responded with a smile.

We followed her through the secured doors into the ER as she continued to make small talk. I knew she could sense the tension and that both Becky and I were worried about what was going on. We followed the triage nurse through the hallway, my hand securely holding Becky's. This was the first time I walked through these hallways as the spouse of a patient, not as an employee. It made me feel somewhat uncomfortable to be on the other side of the spectrum.

Room 11 was one of the largest rooms in the ER. It had large glass doors and was normally used for critical patients, like those that were in cardiac arrest, had a stroke, or had been in a trauma. The whole ER team would fit in this room and the large glass doors would allow the medical staff to keep a constant eye on the patient inside. Becky sat down on the edge of the bed while the nurse handed her a gown.

"That guy over there can help you put this on," she said smiling while her head made a nudging movement into my direction. She left the room closing the curtains along the glass doors to assure privacy.

"Just let them know when you are ready Roy."

"These things are so confusing with the opening to the back," I said, as I helped Becky into her gown. Becky laid down in the bed, and she started to cough immediately. I reached over to the head of the bed and found the lever to release the top part from the bed frame. I squeezed it and, as it made a sudden 'click', it became movable. I continued to pull to raise the head of her bed to a more upright position.

"Let me know when it is high enough sweetie," I said, as I continued to slowly raise the head of the bed.

"That's good," she said, "Thanks babe."

I let go of the lever and the head of the bed stopped moving. I leaned over, landed my lips softly onto hers, and kissed them.

"I love you sweetie."

Her eyes sparkled with joy; her mouth curved to a genuine smile. I sat down on the bed right next to her, holding her hand. A sudden knock on the metal door frame, followed by the curtains being jerked open, as the glass door moved to the side.

"What are you guys doing here?"

It was good to see that our ER nurse was Emily, since she actually knew us both. I worked with her many times, and Becky had met her on many occasions. Emily walked over to the computer screen, flipped the keyboard down from its upright position, swiped her ID across a sensor device, and the computer screen came to life. She asked Becky all kinds of questions about her symptoms, her medical background, her family history, and her current medications. After she finished the computerized intake, she flipped the keyboard back up and swiped her ID once again in front of the sensor to securely lock the computer.

She moved to the corner of the room to the cabinet with all the supplies that she needed to start an IV and draw blood for the lab. I knew the routine; I had done it so many times. I sat back down on the bed, facing Becky. My right hand reached out for hers and she gladly grabbed it as it provided her with a sense of security and stability.

"They are just going to start an IV, draw some blood and give you some fluids to make you feel better, ok sweetie?" Becky nodded with a smile.

The curtains suddenly moved again as Doctor Kawamura stepped into the room. He was average height, probably around 5'10," black hair, brown eyes, normal build, and tanned skin. He had a somewhat complex last name, so most nurses would simply call him doctor K. Upon entering the room, his lips curled to a smile,

"Hey Roy, I did not expect to see you here tonight!"

"You must be Becky," he said as he reached out his right hand towards her. The invitation was not left unanswered, Becky extended her hand to shake his.

"My name is Doctor Kawamura, but most just call me Doctor K. It is nice to meet you."

"Nice to meet you too," Becky responded.

"I work with your husband quite a bit, he is a good man," he said, as their hands let go.

After he completed a wide array of standard questions about her current health situation and her main complaint, he pulled his stethoscope from around his neck, leaned forward closer to Becky, then placed the diaphragm on her back.

"Take a couple of deep breaths in and out for me please," he asked her.

Becky's chest expanded, paused, then decreased in size as she exhaled. Doctor Kawamura kept placing the diaphragm of the stethoscope on different locations on her back to listen to all lung fields. He pulled both earpieces from the stethoscope out from his ears and folded it back around his neck.

"Although you are coughing a lot, your lungs sound pretty clear," he told her.

With a very gentle, calm tone of voice, he explained that he would order a breathing treatment to see if that would help with the cough. He was also going to order a chest X-ray.

"He is nice," Becky said after he left the room.

"Yes, he is," I confirmed with a nod and a smile.

I continued to have that uneasy feeling in the bottom of my stomach. That feeling you have, when you haven't had breakfast for a while and you get really hungry, an almost nauseous feeling. I tried not to display my worries, tried to cover it up, but Becky was too smart, she knew me too well.

"I will be fine babe. Don't worry," she exclaimed with a big smile.

Emily started an IV, drew several tubes of blood, and after she was done, she placed the tubes in a plastic bag with a large biohazard symbol on it and explained that she had to send them off to the lab, but that she would be right back. Within minutes after she left, she walked back into the room, holding a green sheet of paper in her hand that I was very familiar with. It was the official transfer form that we as nurses needed to have, if we were to transfer a patient from the ER to another department, such as the imaging department.

"Okay Becky," she said, "I am going to take you to the X-ray department for a chest X-ray, okay?" Becky raised both her hands up from the bed and gave her two thumbs up.

Emily placed her foot on the big lever at the bottom of the bed. She pushed it down, a loud snapping noise and a small jerking motion confirmed that the wheels were no longer locked. After opening the curtains, I placed my hand on the aluminum frame of the glass sliding door and pushed it to the left. With my right hand placed on the metal bar at the foot end of the bed, I started to pull. Simultaneously, Emily pushed. Out of the room, then a sharp left turn, followed by a ninety-degree right turn, then stopping for the double door that was closed. A quick slap on the large round red button on the wall, and both swung open, one moving inward, the other outward.

We continued our journey and maneuvered Becky's bed through different hallways to the imaging department - radiology. It was not far from the ER. It had four X-ray rooms, two CT scanners, four ultrasound rooms and two interventional rooms for specialized procedures. We started to slow down the bed and Emily instructed me to place it along the hallway wall to the right.

"I will be right back," she said.

She disappeared into the office to the right of us. As she opened the door, I noticed two people sitting behind computers with black and white images on their screens. A collage of bones and joints from different body sections. I reached out to Becky, placed my right hand on her left cheek, leaned over and kissed her lips. No words were spoken, but we both knew. We knew our concerns, our worries, and our fear of the unknown. We both tried to hide it, for the sake of each other.

Emily stepped back out of the room. She pointed to the door right behind us with an oversized '1' in the center.

"We are going into that room, guys."

We moved Becky's bed from the hallway into the X-ray room. In the middle of it was a thin long table, made of hard plastic, no mattress, no pillow, just a sheet. Above the table, in the center, a device that looked like an oversized camera, pointing down at the thin long table. A young female with long blond hair, bundled in a ponytail to the side, was standing behind a safety wall. This lead infused protective barrier was open on one side, so the X-ray technician was able to communicate with the patient, without receiving any radiation from the X-ray machine. She was typing on a keyboard, putting information into the computer system. As we rolled the bed inside the X-ray room, she stepped backward, away from the computer, into the opening of the protective wall.

"Just leave her bed right there," she instructed, "we will do this X-ray in an upright standing position."

One of the benefits of going to a hospital with family members where you work is that you are allowed to stay or even help with certain procedures. Emily made a note on the chart stating: 'Husband Roy is ER nurse here'. As a result, the radiology tech allowed me to stay in the room while she was taking the X-rays. After she was done putting Becky's information into the system, she asked Becky to come out of the bed.

She positioned Becky with her back against a device that was mounted on the wall. The X-ray machine was right in front of her. She helped placing both her hands, with straight arms, on top of the machine. This was done to make sure that nothing would be between the X-ray machine and her chest, obscuring the view. After the tech stepped back behind the safety wall, she instructed me to do the same. When I was standing right behind her, she told Becky,

"Take a deep breath in and hold it!"

Becky's chest expanded to a larger than normal size, at the top of that movement she stopped breathing, holding her breath. A sudden loud clicking noise followed by a hissing sound confirmed the completion of the X-ray.

"Breathe normal," she instructed.

As Becky released the air from her lungs, she immediately started to coughing violently. As if something were stuck in her lungs that wouldn't come out.

"Are you okay?" the X-ray tech asked.

Becky grasped for air and the coughing diminished slowly,

"I am fine," she assured us.

"One more and we will be done," the X-ray tech explained as she walked over to help Becky adjust to a different position.

Every chest X-ray consists of two images, one known as *frontal*, the other is a *lateral* image – from the side. This is done to assure that all areas of the lungs are visible to the radiologist for interpretation.

While the tech was helping Becky, I leaned to my left and tried to get a glance of the X-ray that was just taken. The image was still downloading, and the screen continued to be dark green, nothing there. After the second X-ray was completed, the X-ray tech and helped us getting back to the ER room.

The curtains of ER-room 11 were still open. The TV filled the room with a soft mumbling. Emily and the X-ray tech secured the bed into the same position as before we left. While Emily placed the blood-pressure cuff around Becky's upper arm, the X-ray tech started to place the heart-monitor leads back on Becky's chest. She was holding four cords in her left hand, each cord had a different color: red, black, green, and white. She pulled the protective layer from the sticky side, and as she started to place them in the correct location on Becky's chest, I remembered:

'Smoke over fire, clouds over grass, black over red, white over green'.

The correct placements of the EKG-leads on the chest.

She tapped the screen with her index-finger. It magically turned on and the blood pressure cuff started to make a mechanical sound as it was getting larger around Becky's arm. The cardiac rhythm line suddenly came to life on the screen.

"We will get those x-rays read as soon as possible," the tech explained.

She turned around with one swift movement, like a model showing a new dress, turning around at the end of the runway. She got a hold of the curtains and, as she removed herself from the ER-room, pulled them shut.

The room settled into silence once everyone was gone. Only the soft sound of the TV was noticeable. The ER seemed awkwardly quiet. I spent so many nights here where silence was far from the norm, but tonight, it was one of the very few nights it would have been great to work. Not too many patients, not too much commotion, enough time to provide true patient care for those in need.

Becky was still coughing frequently, but as long as she sat upright, it was noticeably better. I raised myself from the chair and moved towards her bed. Becky smiled, her eyes shimmering like bright little diamonds reflecting in the overhead fluorescent lights. She tapped her left hand on the bed, right next to her, directing me to sit down there. After I sat down, I placed my hand on her knee, our eyes connected, and our smiles synchronized in their motion. Her silence was speaking words of fear and concern. The sudden sound of the curtains being pushed to the side interrupted our togetherness. Doctor Kawamura walked into the room.

There are times when people provide more information by not speaking. Their eyes, their body movements and their postures reveal much more than any word could express. He and I worked many nights together and, when you are down in the trenches with a person, knee-deep in blood, tears, and guts, you learn to read that unspoken language.

As he walked into our room I noticed 'it'. Something was wrong. He stood there at the end of Becky's bed, carefully selecting his words in his head. He knew he had to tread slowly and patiently. He started to explain the results of the chest X-ray. He mentioned two words that I fully understood and never expected to hear tonight: "suspicious appearance."

The chest X-ray revealed a suspicious appearance in the left upper lobe of the left lung. He clarified that nothing was certain until further testing was completed. I knew that tonight was not going to be a short night. On the contrary, it was going to be a long one. Doctor Kawamura continued to explain the next steps that needed to be done, but my mind started to tune out the sound of his voice. I started to realize the massive impact of this ER visit; our lives would never be the same. From this moment on, not hers, not mine, not that of our boys, everything changed in a split second.

This sudden realization caused my stomach to be in a knot, turned upside down, as if it was rammed into a meat grinder, without regret or warning, causing an uncontrollable shiver through my body. The pounding in my chest sounded like drums pacing loudly in my ears, alarming me that my cardiac muscle was working overtime. My oxygen intake became rapid, mental focus fading, turning inward. I wondered how we got here.

My hand on Becky's knee gently clutching, seconds became hours. My mind slowly reclaimed focus, my attention aimed at him. He stood motionless in the middle of the room, staring at us with an aimless and hollow gaze, saying nothing. As my pupils regained more focus, I noticed the uneasiness in his eyes that declared the state of emergency as I was expecting. He knew how bad this was. He knew that I understood the severity of this situation from which almost no escape was possible. Only a few blessed ones were able to avoid the fatal grip of the expected end-result.

Slowly I turned my head as if I were trying not to alert anyone of my movements. My attention towards her, our eyes locked, the room faded, sounds disappeared, just her and I. She was thrown into this mess, unwillingly brand marked. She did not want to be here. She did not belong here. Her pupils sucked me into the depths of her soul, and although no words were spoken, their screams were gruesomely loud. A gentle squeeze from her hand into mine, confirmed our connection, her trust in me, and her fear for what might come her way. A disastrous future lurking from above, like a hawk ready to dive from unknown heights to pierce his claws into his prey, from which no escape was possible; slowly and painfully ripping the life from the helpless victim.

Becky disrupted the silence by asking if this could still be as simple as pneumonia or histoplasmosis. She remained confused about the severity of the situation, pleasantly unaware of the horrific events coming her direction. Or was this a way for her to put it aside, deep down inside, a defense mechanism?

Doctor Kawamura provided us with the proper medical response - that nothing could be diagnosed from an X-ray alone. Further testing was needed to determine the actual severity of the situation. A CT-scan would be more effective in bringing clarity of the possible cause of the 'suspicious appearance'. His eyes showed deep concern and care,

"I think it will be best if we admit you to the hospital so we can complete all necessary testing as soon as possible," he said, "and if we need to do more research, it can be done faster when you are inpatient."

"We might need to do a PET-scan and a biopsy if the CT-scan shows the same problem."

Becky remained soundless, her voice silent, her body motionless. I was aware of her trembling soul inside, I sensed it. Knowingly she placed her fears into the deep dark parts of her subconscious, putting it away deep down and unwilling to give in to the probable outcome of this horrific disaster she was thrown into.

Three

A shimmer of light was creeping from underneath the oversized door. It spread a faint light throughout the room, onto the walls and different objects that were placed here and there. Since my eyes were already adjusted to the darkness, it was easy to detect their shapes; a raised square border on the wall was clearly a picture frame.

Distant sounds from further down the hallway slipped through that same crack between the floor and the door. Sounds of soft voices talking in a friendly conversation, but too far away to understand their words. I aimed my ear toward the direction of the sound, using my auricle as a receiver, trying to find the best angle to amplify the vibrations of sound, but without luck. I was still not able to decipher the words.

The recliner provided by the hospital, for me to sleep on, was almost comfortable. Not sure if it was the lack of sleep or the actual comfort that provided a short, but pleasant rest. Becky was in the hospital bed right next to me. She was still asleep. Her bed was some kind of air mattress, making hissing noises throughout the night. Pumping the mattress up and then systematically letting air out. It was supposed to prevent pressure ulcers.

She was lying on her right side, facing away from me. The outline of her body had a calm rhythm; a gentle raise of her shoulder with a smooth fall. A flow as that of the waves of the ocean, gently rolling on and off the sandy beaches on a calm summer night. It was good to see her resting without a cough.

Earlier, before bed, they gave her some calming medication and that seemed to work well. My eyes flew past her sleeping body towards the digital clock on her nightstand. The green digits provided a soft glare on the top surface of the pinewood bedside table; 04:12am. We arrived in this room about 2am. The admission process to the hospital can take many hours, frequently caused by the meticulous process of paperwork. Since we got this room fairly fast, I knew that the house supervisor or Doctor Kawamura had pulled some strings to speed up the process.

The only hospital rooms available were on the 6th floor, the 'med-surg-floor.' It was called the 'med-surg-floor' because that stands for 'medical-surgery.' All patients that had a procedure done ended up on this floor. Unless the surgery fell under any of the specialties, such as neurosurgery, oncology, and mother-and-baby. Then they would be placed on that specialty floor instead.

Doctor Kawamura wanted to admit Becky to the oncology floor, but there were no more rooms available. Frequently patients would be admitted to the 'med-surg' floor because most of them would be short-term hospital stays.

We got the bigger suite that was located at the end of the hallway. The end-rooms, also known as the 'suites' are just a little nicer and bigger than the normal rooms.

I glared at the ceiling, motionless, not really focusing on anything, just a numb blank gaze. From the moment I received Lisa's call earlier this evening when I was at work, I had one mission on my mind: to take care of my Becky. As an ER-nurse and Paramedic, I followed my trained instincts to provide the best possible outcome for those I was taking care of. There is not much time for emotion at that stage, there is only time for doing. Saving lives, providing care, and giving the right medications. To assure the best possible outcome for those

I cared for. This time, it was not a stranger, but my own sweetheart. That made things just a little more complicated.

Now, finally, I allowed myself time to think, to grant emotions onto the stage. The different events that happened last night passed by my conscious mind as I analyzed each event individually. As I was laying there, wrapped in the darkness of the room, I already knew the diagnosis of tonight's discovery. I knew that the 'suspicious appearance' of that mass would only allow for one possible result. The only question remaining was how bad was it? If it was only in the lung, surgery could take care of it, but if it had already spread through her body, not much could be done besides chemotherapy.

Pressure started to build in my chest, flowing up towards my throat. My eyes swelled, a small tear fell from my right eye, trailing down my temporal into the hairline where it got stuck. Another one escaped, now from the other eye, it pooled between my eye and the bridge of my nose. I placed my finger into the puddle to wipe it dry. I wanted to cry out loud, I needed Becky's arm around me for comfort, but I swallowed my pain, I could not give in, I had to stay strong for her.

I can't say anything, I told myself.

I had to stay quiet, to not reveal any of my thoughts, until proven by biopsy.

I broke my gaze away from the ceiling. Moved my body around onto my other side. I needed to get some more sleep.

God only knows how long it will be before they wake us, I thought as I started to force myself to sleep. They always wake you up at ungodly hours. I understand that most physicians will do their rounds in the hospital real early, before they have clinic, but why not do all their labs later in the morning?

I softly placed my left hand on Becky's bed, not touching her, but knowing she was there. The pattern of her breathing was a soothing rhythm that caused a calmness which allowed me to close my eyes and let go of the day. My breathing became deep and slow, I allowed the darkness to take control, I sensed a falling sensation, I did not resist.

A sudden blast of bright light burst into the room, caused by the opening of the large door by the floor nurse, resulting in a rude awakening from a short slumber. My eyes ripped open, causing an instant burning sensation created by the lack of sleep. I tried to focus on the alarm to determine what time it was, but before I could register the numbers on the display, a joyful voice declared,

"Good morning! It is six o'clock! Time to get ready!"

My brain was cramping, causing a headache, as if I had been partying too long the night before. Becky opened her eyes unwillingly, and although she did not say anything, I knew she must be feeling the same. I pushed myself up on the recliner, leaned over toward Becky, and as she started to lean toward me, I whispered,

"Good morning babe," right before our lips connected for a brief moment.

"Morning sweetie," she replied.

"After your morning labs and vital signs," the nurse said, "you are expected down at imaging for an 8 o'clock PET-scan."

This nurse had way too much enthusiasm for this early in the morning.

"After that, you will be back here on the floor for lunch. Then later this afternoon you are expected at interventional radiology for a biopsy."

It was obvious that someone had been busy overnight to arrange for both these tests to be done so quickly. Normally it would take at least 24 to 48 hours to get one or both tests scheduled. This was unexpectedly fast. Although never confirmed nor denied, I assumed certain influence from an ER-doc assured the quick testing. I reached my hand out to Becky's, and as it found hers, we interlocked our fingers.

"That's good babe," I said, "let's get all this testing out of the way as soon as possible."

Her eyes screamed fear, a painful loud cry for help, but her voice remained calm.

"It could still be just pneumonia, right?" she asked, "Or that histoplasmosis disease Lisa was talking about?"

Since we had about twenty chickens on our land, Lisa did some research on lung diseases when Becky continued to cough so much. Histoplasmosis had come up several times. It can be caused by inhalation of a fungus frequently found in bird droppings. Lisa made the connection that having chickens and cleaning the chicken coop could have caused the histoplasmosis. A possibility for sure, but the results from the x-ray and CT-scan pointed to a more disastrous cause for the cough and fatigue.

The floor-nurse rolled in a tall cart with a monitor attached to it. A small basket attached to the front was holding a blood pressure cuff with tubing, a pulse oximetry device, and a thermometer was attached to the side. One of the wheels was making an irritating squeaking noise while it was making weird circles in all directions, like it had a mind on its own.

While in the process of securing the blood-pressure cuff around Becky's upper arm, she explained that the lab tech would stop by later to draw some blood. She pushed a large green button on the right side of the monitor and the screen lit up, making a single beeping sound. A sudden machine-like hissing sound caused the blood pressure cuff to inflate and enlarge in size. Simultaneously, the pulse oximetry device was placed on Becky's index finger. The thermometer was swiped along her forehead, passing down the right-side of her face, moving past the ear toward her neck.

As the blood pressure cuff started to reach its maximum capacity, the hissing sound became tight, more difficult, followed by a slow release of air. Suddenly, the monitor displayed numbers that represented Becky's temperature, her blood pressure and the actual oxygen levels in her blood.

"All your vitals are looking good," the floor-nurse explained.

She unwrapped the cuff from Becky's arm, placed it back in the basket together with the pulse-ox device. Then disappeared into the hallway while dragging the cart with her, like a mother hauling a small, unwilling, and screaming child through the grocery store.

I stood up from the recliner, walked around the end of the bed and sat down next to Becky, facing her. She grabbed my hand, folded her fingers around it and asked,

"So, what exactly are they going to do?"

I realized that the medical world and the terminology used can be extremely confusing for those who do not work in this field. I started to explain,

"A PET-scan is almost the same as a normal CT-scan. The only difference is that they will inject you with a radioactive glucose to see if there is any activity."

"Okay... and then what?" she asked.

"If there is increased activity at certain areas, that will be a concern and they will want to do a biopsy to see what it is."

I tried to be as careful as possible with my word choice. Even though I had a very strong feeling the 'suspicious appearance' was cancer, until there was a positive PET-scan with a positive biopsy, no one would really know for sure. There was no reason to have Becky all worried in case it turned out to be nothing.

I think she knew and understood what was going on. She was well aware of that potential outcome of cancer, even though she continued with the possibility of pneumonia or the 'chicken disease', like she called it. I think she was not ready to face it yet. She had to get there on her own terms, at her own pace, at her time, whenever she was ready for it. I knew and I understood all too well.

"Let's call the boys real quick before they go to Kids Club," she suggested.

Last night I talked to Lisa to tell her about the admission to the hospital. Without any hesitation, she offered to stay with the boys as long as was needed and that she would get them to and from Kids Club. Becky dialed her number. Within a few rings, Lisa responded,

"I have two boys here that want to talk to their mama and papa!"

Becky's eyes lit up and her smile filled the room as she was talking to Connor and Dane. These two little guys were her absolute everything.

"They are just going to figure out why mama has such a bad cough ok? We will be back home before you know it," she told them.

I could hear the boys just being all wild and crazy on the other side of the line. Lisa put the phone on speaker so they could both talk to Becky at the same time. They were typical young boys; rowdy and loud.

"I love you guys," Becky shouted.

"Love you Mama," both boys yelled back, almost at the same time.

Lisa came back on and offered to pick them up from Kids Club also, since she was off from work anyway.

"Let me know what's going on guys," she asked.

The hospital bathroom was barely big enough for one person. The extra-large shower area, with railings attached to the walls for support of patients, absorbed most of the space available. Right above the small oval-shaped sink, a square mirror. I looked at my own reflection. The short night left its toll; dark bags, red eyes, wild hair. I turned on the faucet, cold water only. I leaned forward, collected as much water as I could in my cupped hands. Right before I splashed it onto my face, I held my breath. The cold shock provided an unexpected refreshing result. Again, and again, splashing water to my face, trying to wash away the shortness of the night.

With both my eyes closed, I reached for the towel hanging somewhere to right of the sink. Unaware of the exact location, I hit the wall with an open hand. Slowly moving it down the wall, tapping it softly, as if the sounding of the wall would provide me with information about the correct location of the towel. As if I had the same capabilities of a bat and his sonar system. My hand found a soft resistance, it was the towel I was looking for. Like a grab-hook that found its prize, I folded my fingers around it and pulled it toward me.

I wiped the skin of my face dry, pressing hard as if I was pulling off an old face to reveal a new one. I still felt that pit in my stomach. Upset and nauseous from missing breakfast, or just miserable from not enough sleep? Maybe both. Before my mind could wander off too much, three loud knocks on the door pulled my drifting mind back into reality. The door slowly moved inwards, followed by a soft voice,

"Transport here," a kind female voice announced, "I am here to take you to your PET-scan."

A young female in her mid-twenties with a gentle and friendly appearance walked in. Right away she started to move some things around, for her to be able to roll the bed out of the room. She secured both bedside railings in an upward position and placed several blankets around Becky's body and explained,

"The hallways are always cold so I brought you some extra blankets."

Becky smiled and confirmed she was comfortable. The extra-wide doors provided plenty of space for the bed to go through. As we started to move out of the room and into the hallway, I walked beside the bed, my left arm stretched out, holding hands with my sweetheart, as if we were just strolling along the beach on a beautiful sunny day.

After the elevator ride down, a labyrinth of different hallways guided us to the PET-scan area. The friendly transport lady, who chatted the whole way, parked the bed on the right side of the hallway with remarkable precision. She explained that she would inform 'them' of our arrival and disappeared through a door to the right with a large sign stating 'Employees Only'. Within minutes another female came out.

"You must be Becky, right?" she asked.

Becky nodded to confirm that assumption. The tech introduced herself as she started to move Becky's bed towards the double doors that were positioned right in front of us. She looked at me and asked me to come along. The procedure room was immediately to the right of the double doors. The scanner was shaped like a giant donut and placed in the middle of the room. It made a soft humming noise. A thin long bed, without a mattress, was placed in the middle of the hole of the scanner.

A male tech came out to greet us and helped Becky from her bed to the scanner table. He started to explain the scan procedure to Becky, when the female tech asked me to follow her out. Before doing so, I walked over to Becky, leaned towards her, excused myself to the male tech, and kissed Becky's cheek.

"You will be fine babe. I will be right outside here, waiting for you ok?"

"Okay," she softly responded.

Her appearance on the outside may have been calm, but on the inside, I knew she was screaming for help. Scared for what was going to happen, troubled over the possible outcome, afraid for the future. I placed my hand on her face, another soft kiss, now on her tender lips and I whispered, as if I was telling her a secret,

"I love you sweetie."

Her eyes were tender, her smile soft.

I walked toward the door, out from the scanning room, where the female tech was waiting for me. The voice of the male tech faded away as I started to increase the distance between him and me. I knew he was giving Becky instructions about the scan. I knew he was also trying to ease her.

The female tech was standing in front of a console filled with screens, knobs, switches, and several keyboards. Her fingers rapidly tapped on a keyboard as she stared at a screen. Without looking up, she stated,

"You must be Roy, right? From the ER?"

I turned my head towards her, slightly tilted, my eyes scanning her appearance, trying to recall her from my memory bank. Before I was able to summon any memory of her, she explained,

"I picked up a couple of your patients, one time, when you were working in the ER. Also, Emily told me that you were coming."

The male tech interrupted our conversation, "Okay, we are good to go."

The female tech pushed several buttons causing the CT-scanner to come alive. The increasing humming sound was even noticeable here in the control room, behind the thick glass wall.

An outline of Becky's body appeared on the middle screen, one as you would normally see on a regular CT scan. Suddenly the picture started to display shades of red, yellow, and orange. The female tech pointed to the one which was the largest, the left upper lobe of Becky's left lung. It was bright red with some orange shading around it.

"This red color means that there is a lot of uptake of radioactive glucose," she explained.

"Increased uptake is most likely cancer," she added.

My eyes examined the images on the computer screen. The amount of the red spots inside her body made my heart sink. My soul started to suffocate in sorrow and misery, barely able to breath. I was being dragged down by an immense amount of weight, deep down to the miseries of hell. So many areas lit up. Her left lung, her hips, throughout her chest, and along many vertebrae of her spine. My eyes were glued to the screen, as if I were being hypnotized. I wanted to scream at the top of my lungs, but my lips remained silent. The female tech, observing the same disastrous images, tried to make things seem less horrible.

"Nothing is sure until they do a biopsy," she explained.

She was using a technique we also use in the ER; trying to keep things neutral, and let the specialist bring the bad news. I did not fall for it. I was looking at the same scan. I could see. I knew what was going on. I had too much information, and too much medical training. Everything was leading to the same diagnosis: cancer. It had most likely started in the left lung, with many metastases now throughout her whole body.

It didn't take long for the scan to be completed. The female tech and I walked back into the scanning room. Becky was patiently lying still on the CT table that was too hard for comfort. The tech told Becky that the scan was done, and that the results would come later that morning, after it was analyzed by a radiologist. I was relieved to hear that she informed Becky about the delay in results. Although I was aware of the horrific situation that was going to unfold in the near future, I still had a glimmer of hope that the biopsy results could be negative. No matter what, I would rather not be the one who had to deliver this horrific and heart wrenching news to any person, especially if that person was so close to my heart.

The tech decided not to wait for transport and brought us back to the room herself. I held Becky's hand on the way back, just as I had earlier that morning.

***

Becky and I met on Thursday May 28, 1998. I was still working as a roofer at that time. A friend of mine called me that afternoon to see if I wanted to come over for a drink in the evening at our favorite bar in town: the 'Blues on Grand'. Normally I am always up for a drink with him, but this time I was too tired. He was persistent in his quest so finally I gave in and told him I would be there around 8:30pm.

I remember walking into the bar. The smoke from cigarettes instantly burned my eyes, the distinct stench of tobacco penetrated my nostrils, clouds of smoke lingered like morning mist. The live blues music was so loud you could barely hear a word unless someone was yelling right into your ear.

I noticed my friend sitting at a small round table with two ladies. The moment he saw me, he walked over with a big smile on his face, glad to see me. His right hand landed on my left shoulder, he pulled me close. Leaning forward, I turned my head so my right ear would have the best angle to absorb his voice. He explained that he ran into his hairstylist earlier, and that she was here with a friend. He then pulled me along, towards the table, and on top of his lungs, he introduced both ladies.

"This is Sally," he shouted, while pointing at a dark-haired female.

I waved my right hand to say 'Hi'.

"... and this is Becky!"

She was wearing a white fluffy sweater, bright blonde curly hair. Her eyes, bright green like radiant emeralds sparkling beautifully in the dark smoky bar. Despite my resistance, I was being pulled in. I could not resist.

Becky always told me, or anyone who wanted to hear the story, that she would never forget that first moment. She always assumed that she would grow old single, no husband, no kids, only cats, many cats. She would be known as the crazy old cat lady from the corner. She would make it clear that it all changed that night. That night, at the 'Blues on Grand' when 'the crazy Dutchman' stepped into her life.

Even though I would always feel some selfish pride when she would convey her story to friends and family, she never realized that it was her who changed my life. She was the one that allowed me to walk beside her, I was the one blessed.

Her eyes trapped me inside her soul from which there was no escape. I surrendered my existence to her willingly and became her prisoner for life, with pleasure.

***

Although the interventional radiology room was dark, the low glow, caused by the many monitors and equipment, providing enough light to see. Several machines were humming, clarifying they were ready to start doing whatever they were supposed to do. The radiology nurse was talking to Becky while helping her onto the hard procedure table. I stood right next to Becky, ready to assist if needed.

A tall skinny man stood up from behind the desk and walked towards us. I recognized him; it was Doctor Cook. He was the interventional radiologist that I worked with many times while working in the ER. He greeted me with a smile, reaching his hand out to me. We connected with a short but warm handshake. His left hand landed simultaneously on my shoulder.

"Roy," he said, "this is your wife?"

"Yes, she is," I confirmed.

He turned around with a swift move, introduced himself to Becky, then started to walk towards the desk area where he had come from. He gestured me to follow him. I turned my head to Becky where she was still being assisted by the nurse.

"I am going to talk to Doctor Cook really quick," I said, "I will be right here babe."

Her right hand raised up from the bed. A thumb up signaled me that she was good.

I walked over to where Doctor Cook was sitting and stood right beside him as he was analyzing the PET-scan from earlier that day.

"As you can see on this image," while he was placing the tip of his pen at a bright red area on Becky's right hip bone,

"This would be the best location to get the biopsy from, not the supraclavicular lymph node."

He turned his chair around and stopped, with precise accuracy, right in front of me. He raised himself out from the chair and continued,

"Initially they instructed me to obtain a biopsy from the left supraclavicular lymph node, but I believe it is best to go for the area that is furthest away from the possible initial mass."

Suddenly, he changed his voice to a more gentle, soft, caring tone. His eyes exhibited a concern I had not seen in him before. It revealed a caring that is rare to find, especially in healthcare. Too often we become numb to individual cases because we are consistently exposed to pain, disaster, hurt, and death. Causing us healthcare professionals to frequently assume a more neutral standpoint to, ultimately, protect ourselves.

As he walked with me, away from the procedure area, he explained,

"Roy, your wife is really sick. These images from the PET-scan, you have seen them ... I am sorry man ... it does not look good."

From the bottom of my stomach, a sensation of powerlessness was creeping up from deep down below, slowly taking over my existence, as if someone injected me with a drug that I didn't want but was leisurely crawling through my veins to occupy every cellular structure inside my body. I stood there alone, in the middle of the room. I could hear muffled voices, noticing people moving around as shadows. I zoned out the surrounding sounds and movements. My eyes slowly turned towards Becky; she was laying on the procedure table. My soul reached out to hers. She was not yet aware of what was coming.

We had been back in the room now for several hours. Becky was still a little drunken from the sedation she received for the procedure earlier in the afternoon. The silence caused my mind to wander off. It was going 100,000 miles an hour and I could not slow it down as I thought about treatment options that could deal with the likely diagnosis of cancer. Although I worked in the medical field, in which conventional treatment was the norm, I also believe in natural and holistic healing options.

I am convinced that my raising in the Netherlands and my exposure to holistic and homeopathic treatment plans there, caused my inborn conviction of the power of natural healing. Natural, homeopathic, and other alternative healing methods are widely accepted and used in the Netherlands. I believe that our bodies are capable of fighting off most diseases themselves, as long as we provide it with healthy and proper nutrition. Chemotherapy, radiation, and surgery are not the only options.

When I still lived in the Netherlands, I remember that there was a lot of commotion about a diet that was developed by the Dutch doctor Cornelis Moerman, known as the *Moerman Diet*. This doctor believed that there was a relationship between nutrition and cancer, and that with the right diet, our body would be able to fight off cancer. Some found it to be worthwhile information, while others found it to be quackery. This was going on back in the 1970s-1980s.

Over the last two decades, science and research have proven that a good and healthy nutritional intake can keep us stay healthy and free from disease. It will also assist in a strong immune system that allows our bodies to fight off or battle any disease. The newest development in the treatment of certain cancers are injections to boost the immune system to have our own bodies, our own immune system, battle the cancer instead of using conventional chemotherapy or radiation.

I wondered why some will only follow conventional treatment plans. Why not research all options? Why not use all the knowledge we have available from all over the world? Why only listen to medical doctors?

I was going to research medical approaches, what other countries offer for cancer treatment, and what natural healing plans were available. I made it my mission to research everything, then find the best options and make them work together.

Suddenly, unexpectedly, my thoughts were disrupted. From the corner of my eyes, I noticed a person standing outside of the room. He was flipping through the pages of Becky's binder. Every patient that was admitted to the hospital had a binder in which results, orders, and treatment plans were noted. I could only see the backside of his white coat, but when he turned towards the room, I recognized his face. Doctor Bryon Johnson from the Chest Infectious Diseases group.

I had seen him before in the FR, but never had the pleasure of working with him. He stood in front of the open door, and although he was looking straight at me, he maintained the courtesy of knocking on the doorpost to announce his appearance.

By this time, Becky was up and awake. She was sitting straight up in bed, her legs pulled up to her chest with her arms folded around them. Doctor Johnson walked in and introduced himself, pulled up a chair to the side of Becky's bed, and sat down. He started to summarize in detail about his interpretation of the numerous X-rays, CT-scans, and PET-scan.

"The only thing we are still waiting for are the results of the biopsy," he explained while alternating his attention between the both of us.

Becky started to lean forward, placed her chin on top of her knees. She took a deep breath in, held it, and as she let it go, she asked hopeful,

" ... but it could still be pneumonia, right?"

He leaned back, placed his right hand on his chin. His thumb and index-finger started to stroke it in a slow deliberate motion. His eyes started to have a sudden increase in glitter. I realized that he started to tear up, as he understood the severity of the situation.

"Becky, you are very sick. The chance for this to be pneumonia is slim, very slim..."

Becky sighed, no words escaped from her lips, but her body spoke loudly; her shoulders lowered slightly, her facial tone grim.

"We will know for sure late Thursday or early Friday if this growth is cancer or not, but for now I will contact oncology for a referral," he explained.

Two words that had not been spoken yet were now placed on the table, 'cancer' and 'oncology.' The silence was disturbing. Becky's gaze faded, her breath deep and slow. Doctor Johnson placed both his hands on his knees, leaned forward to raise himself to standing.

"It will be best to stay here at the hospital until the results are complete," he continued, "one of my colleagues will be coming by tomorrow or Friday."

Slowly he turned around and disappeared from the room. Becky's silence was agonizing.

The vibration of my phone broke the muteness. My screen displayed *Lisa Mobile.* My eyes went from the screen back to Becky, her eyes were locked on to mine, her sadness was dimming her beautiful radiant being.

"It is probably the boys," I said.

"Let's not say anything until the biopsy is back," Becky responded.

I nodded.

Lisa explained that she had taken time off from work until she was no longer needed to take care of the boys. I told her about the events that happened, but that I was planning on coming home tomorrow to pick up the boys from Kids Club myself. Becky and I both decided that it was important for me to spend some time with them to allow for some normalcy in their lives.

"I will get the boys on the phone, so Becky can talk to them," Lisa said.

I placed the phone in Becky's hand, her mood improved instantly. Her boys were her love and her life. She started talking with them as if nothing was going on. She explained that she was still in the hospital because they were still trying to figure out why she was coughing so much.

Even after she ended the phone call, her eyes were still on fire from excitement. All the issues and worries of the day disappeared as snow from the sun. Her hands were flying all over the place, as if she were painting an abstract piece of art on a large canvas, while she told me all about Connor and Dane.

It was a joy to see her so happy. She radiated pleasure; it was an unexpected but welcomed change for this day. Just for a short time, we both forgot all negativity, it was a good pause for a moment.

Four

A loud bashing on the door, followed by full bright light caused by a simple flip of a light switch, rudely interrupted my superficial sleep. Hospital recliners do not provide any support for those with lower back problems, and do not offer comfortable sleeping options. The nights at the hospital were short, with many waking moments caused by the consistent tossing and turning while in pursuit of getting comfortable for much needed rest. The military style roll calls in the mornings were not welcomed and always too early.

My eyelids ripped open after the morning call from the nurse. My right hand tapped on the side of the recliner, trying to find the handle that would allow it to come back into an upright position. After I got a hold of the lever, I pushed down hard and the backrest came back up while simultaneously the footrest went down. Becky was wide awake and seemed to have had a good night of sleep.

"Morning, sweetie," she said with a smile.

I wrestled myself out of the recliner, leaned towards her. She placed her hand on my face, followed by a short, but meaningful kiss that was filled with tenderness and love.

"Good morning babe," I responded.

I stepped into the galley, just three doors down from Becky's room, searching for some much-needed caffeine. The smell of old, dried-up, highly concentrated coffee that had been standing on the warmer all night penetrated my nostrils. It caused a resistance in me to even try to drink this concoction of water and caffeine that was trapped in a dark stained-glass jar. I fought through the repulsive odor and poured the black tar-like substance into a Styrofoam cup, dumped two sweetener packages in it, and although I normally never use any creamer, I decided to pour a large amount into the substance, to ease the flavor. I raised the cup towards my lips, holding my breath, and carefully sipped. It was warm and somewhat resembled coffee. Although the revolting smell was overwhelming, it was what I needed to jumpstart my senses.

I scavenged through several drawers in search of some crackers, particularly sweet graham crackers. Those crackers, utilized as a spoon to scoop peanut butter from a small plastic cup, are the best hospital snack you can get. Working night shifts in the ER will teach you to consume this combination to maintain the stomach growling to a minimum. Triumphantly, I held my treasure of cupped black tar in one hand and four graham crackers with two peanut butter cups in the other. I walked through the hallway back to Becky's room. I planted myself back in the recliner and devoured the goodies in a minimum amount of time.

"How is your breakfast babe?" Becky asked with a sarcastic smirk.

With my mouth full, I looked up, smiled, and gave her a thumbs up.

She cracked up, laughed, her eyes shined, "Glad you are enjoying it."

I swallowed the sticky mixture, sipped the thickened coffee, and enlightened her about the addiction that most ER night staffers have to graham crackers with peanut butter. She slowly shook her head and smiled.

Last night we decided that I would go home today. Although I wanted to stay in the hospital with her, it was important to keep some normalcy for the boys. I would come back later that night and also bring some clean clothes for Becky.

The drive home was a welcome change of scenery. The morning sun was bright but left the air delightfully cool. It could be the beginning of one of those smothering hot summer days, but right now it was a pleasure to be outside. The car seat felt comfortable, it provided better support than the hospital recliner. I cracked my window open to get some fresh air on my face. It gave me some clarity and well needed non-hospital air. I had just gotten off the phone with Lisa and she had explained that she dropped the boys off at Kids Club earlier that morning and that she would be back at the house around five. As I ended the phone call, I realized what a wonderful friend she was; helpful, unselfish, willing to be there at all times if possible, and the boys loved her to pieces.

The warm water poured down on my head. A million raindrops making rhythmic sounds, causing my eyes to close shut and fade away. Rivers of liquid warmth flowed down over my face, gently falling along my sides and my back, caressing my body. The warm friendliness of these streams was comforting and sucked out the stress and worries from my abused body. Tension and burden were pulled out and drowned in the water to be flushed away down the drain. I stood there motionless, with my eyes closed, numb and mindless. The warm flows of water wrapped around me as a blanket, providing the relaxation I needed. Just a short moment of no pain, no worries, no nothing; just me and the comfort of warm relief, quietness and peace. This little break from the hospital was much needed for my mental sanity.

The smell of freshly brewed coffee was liberating. The house was filled with its odor, providing me with a feeling of home comfort. I sat down at our wood dining room table. My right hand folded around the cup, and as I brought it to my lips, it was joined midway for support by the other hand. The rim of the cup reached my lips, a long slow breeze flew past my lips onto the surface of the hot liquid to cool it down. The first sip of this warm blackness, gently flowing down my throat, provided the expected comfort inside my body. As I sipped small amounts of coffee, my eyes aimed at my laptop, sitting on the table, right in front of me. A soft buzzing sound, and a bright screen staring at me, patiently awaiting my orders. I placed the cup of goodness on the table next to the laptop, then positioned my fingers on top of the keys to start my research.

As I started to type, the keys made soft clicking sounds.

'Moerman therapy Netherlands.'

A variety of responses appeared on the screen. I folded my hands together in front of my face, creating a resting place for my chin. My eyes shifted from left to right, absorbing the data. I moved the cursor to the selection I needed, and with a small tap of my right index finger on the mouse, the screen changed and a new page of information appeared. It was the 'Moerman Association' page written in Dutch. Easy for me, but for those that are unfamiliar with this language, it would be impossible to analyze.

With my research into the 'Moerman diet' many other websites appeared on the screen. Each one of them were pulling at me for more attention; they all needed to be researched. From the 'Gerson therapy' that had a similar approach as the 'Moerman therapy', to juicing, to vitamin-C infusions, green diets, and so on. The list seemed limitless. For every therapy or option, there were opposing views and opinions. People who had bad experiences with one or the other because they did not receive the expected result, thus called it quackery. Others praised these types of therapies and reported amazing healing stories. I read each research article in great detail, absorbing more and more information about all the different holistic and natural approaches for the treatment of cancer.

I leaned back, stretched my arms out towards the ceiling, opening and closing my hands as if I was grabbing the air. I moved my shoulder blades closer to each other and released a soft growl. As my arms moved back towards the keyboard, I noticed my watch. It was almost four o'clock. I had lost complete track of time.

"Holy mother of God," I yelled out loud.

I jumped out of the chair as if I were sitting on a hot stove. I knew I only had fifteen minutes to get to Kids Club to pick up Connor and Dane. I had spent over six hours researching.

I parked my truck in the parking lot, right next to the elementary school where Kids Club was being held. Kids club was a summer program for children from kindergarten to high school. I arrived on time, but the children were not back yet. Today was pool day and the Kids Club busses would transport them to the city pool and back. Since the busses were not in the parking lot, I knew they were still on their way back.

I relaxed my hands on the steering wheel, radio off, air-conditioning blasting cold air into my face, providing a revitalizing breeze. My eyes zoomed into nothing, just a blank gaze, my brain turned off. Tuesday was just a short time ago yet felt so far away. So much had happened in the last 48 hours. The painful facts were undeniable. There was no need for a biopsy report to confirm the actual diagnosis. I realized that postponing it might be a technique to allow the patient to accept a verdict that no one wants to hear.

Cancer has no prejudice, no regrets, no preferences. It is not racist, nor does it care about your bank account. It strikes, randomly;

some live to tell, some don't. My focus was not on the 'why' but on the 'what now.'

I was not occupied with the reason, nor was I seeking justification. My mission was set, clear as daylight: Becky will live, cancer free. We will find a way. We will find a cure. She will be one of those miracles that was given up on by the medical world, but her cancer would soon be no longer detectable. This was my duty, my assignment, my quest; and I would do whatever it would take to assure that outcome.

Three Kids Club busses arrived at the side entrance. As they pulled up, the side-doors glided open and flows of children were streaming through it, like fish escaping from the nets of fishermen. Crowds of children ran towards the entrance of the school, guided by adults that were strategically positioned along the sidewalks. Their main job was to control the flow of youngsters and provide safety. Through the flocks of small human beings, I saw two familiar faces. Connor and Dane were running with all the others towards the school. They were not paying attention to anything, too busy having loud conversations with their friends, swinging their arms all over, laughing and talking.

An uncontrollable excitement welled up inside my chest. Although it had been only a few days since I had last seen them, it felt like an eternity. The feeling rushed up to my face, my eyes slowly filling with tears. I opened the door and got out of the truck. I was ready to run over to them, but as soon as I stepped out, Connor beat me to it. He suddenly saw me, stopped, grabbed Dane by his arm and yelled,

"There is Papa!" Both started running towards me, screaming,

"Papa!! … Papa!!"

One of the adults that was corralling the kids, recognized me and allowed the boys to break free. Connor was the first to arrive, faster than lighting. The last couple of feet he jumped, flying through the air like a condor. While he was in mid-air, I caught him and he landed right in my arms.

"Papa!" was all he could bring out as he squeezed his little face against my body, locking his arms around me.

Dane's little legs were going as fast as he could run, just a few seconds behind Connor. Moments after Connor latched on, Dane was there.

"Papa!! Papa!!" he exclaimed at the top of his lungs.

His body landed right next to Connor's. Both boys entrapped me, each from one side. My arms surrounded them. I pulled them close to me, kissing their heads, from one to the other and back.

"Hey guys, how are you? I missed you both so much."

I was fighting back my tears, but a few escaped from their prison and gently landed on their soft hair. Unaware of the delivery of the drops of joy, they both started to ramble on about their day, how excited they were to see me, and the fun time they were having with Lisa. I opened the backdoor of my truck and they climbed in like little monkeys, talking my ears off.

I knew most of the parents that were there to pick up their kids. Several of them waved at us, and as I waved back to them, I realized that none of them were even remotely aware of the disaster our family was in. None of them knew about Becky's upcoming shattering diagnosis and what kind of impact that would have on our family for the rest of our lives.

The boys jumped out of the truck when we arrived at home, running to the front door and burst inside the house. I followed them at a much slower pace. I closed the door behind me and walked up the stairs to the living room. I found my chair, lowered myself into the soft cushion and leaned back. I pulled my phone from my jeans pocket, unlocked the screen, and called Becky. She answered the call within just a couple of rings.

"Hi babe. How are you doing?" she asked.

As I started to explain that it was good to be home for a little bit and to take a real shower, both boys ran into the living room. They must have heard me talking on the phone.

"I will talk to you later babe," I said, "when I get back around five. Here are the boys." I blew a kiss through the phone, then handed it over to Connor.

He talked about his day and walked towards the loveseat to sit down. Dane was sitting next to him, anxious to talk to her, but waiting patiently until Connor was done. After a colorful description of his day, Connor placed his lips on the bottom of the phone and kissed it,

"I love you Mama! See you soon!" Then handed the phone to Dane, leaned back and was quiet.

As Dane was talking away about his day, I could hear Becky's voice responding. She sounded so excited and happy to just talk to them both. Connor stayed seated on the couch, staring at Dane with his big beautiful eyes and a big smile. He was making sure his little brother was doing fine.

***

When Becky and I met, we were both in our mid-30's. We got married on February 24, 1999 and later that summer she said she wanted kids. Becky became pregnant with our first child, Connor, in

December that year. Not long after Connor was born, she suddenly said while we were out for dinner on one of our date-nights,

"I think we should give Connor a brother or a sister."

She explained that she always enjoyed her time with her brother and sisters and that we should not take that pleasure away from Connor. Dane was born in December 2001, a short sixteen months after Connor. Although they were close in age, at this particular moment, while Dane was sitting there, excited, talking to his mom on the phone while she was in the hospital, I detected the 'big brother' in Connor. He was concerned about his younger brother and felt the need to ensure that he was ok.

***

The hospital parking lot was packed. It was a good thing that I could park in employee parking. It was about 5:15pm and as usual, this was a busy time. Many people were getting off work and would stop by to see their loved ones in the hospital. I entered through the employee entrance on the east side of the building. It felt weird. I was not in scrubs and I did not come to work. Instead, I was wearing jeans and a t-shirt. I was a visitor. As I passed the nurses station, the charge nurse, Shari, was sitting at her desk. She looked up and welcomed me with a smile.

"How are you doing buddy?" she asked.

Shari is a gentle person with a big heart and she spread kindness like only a few select people can. She is genuinely gifted in the caring for others, and as I looked at her, I let that question soak in. My face became grim, pressing my lips together because they started to quiver uncontrollably, my eyes filled up with tears. I placed my hand over my mouth as if I wanted to cover up my sadness. As I responded in a vibrating voice, words came out cracking, I could no longer resist my need to let go. Tears flew along both my cheeks, my shoulders shaking,

"It really sucks," was all I could say.

It came from the bottom of my soul. It was buried deep down inside me, but I felt comfortable enough around her to tell the truth. She stood up from her chair, folded her arm around me, as a caring mother would comfort her child. She walked me over to the 'patient private room' and closed the door as we walked in. She sat right in front of me, her hands holding mine, not saying anything. She was just there to listen, to hold, to comfort.

An uncontrollable flow of emotions was streaming from my eyes, my shoulders shrugging. I let go of the urge to be the strong one, the tough one. Tears continued to come, streaming along my face. She just squeezed my hand.

"It's okay buddy, it's okay," she gently whispered.

The last 48 hours consisted of a continuous flow of horrific and devastating information. Test after test with negative results kept beating us down. It was as if someone was hitting me with a baseball bat, violently, consistently, pounding me, harder and harder. I could not show Becky my pain, I needed to be strong for her. I needed to be her rock in this unfair, wild ocean that was trying to drag us down into the depths of despair. I needed to be strong for her and our boys. Only for the select few that I trusted could I show my pain, my fears, my tears. Shari allowed me to have an outburst of pain and emotion. It was between her and I. No one, especially not Becky nor the boys, would know.

Instead of taking the overcrowded elevator, I decided to take the stairs. For one, it would take forever to get to the sixth floor because it would probably stop at every level. But more importantly, I did not want anyone to notice the redness in my eyes. Besides, I needed the exercise anyway.

I reached the med-surg floor without too many problems. I grabbed the metal handle of the heavy fire-door and pulled it towards me. There was a large window to the left and I decided to catch my breath for a moment and just stare outside. A few minutes of absolute silence passed. Silence of sound, silence of mind, just a blank stare into nothingness allowed me to regain control and posture.

A soft but noticeable 'ping' announced the arrival of the elevator. The doors slid open and as several people stepped from the elevator onto the floor, I decided it was time for me to move. I turned around, my shoes made a delicate squeaking sound, past the elevators, and made two left turns into the long hallway towards Becky's room.

Her door was cracked open and I could hear multiple voices talking. I placed my hand in the middle of the cold steel door, pushed, and it moved inward without any resistance. Becky was sitting in the bed, upright, with her legs folded underneath her. Although I barely made a sound, she immediately turned her head toward me when I walked in. She smiled; her eyes sparkled bright. She raised both arms up, holding them out towards me.

"Hey babe," she said as she made the 'come here' signal with both her hands.

I stepped towards her and leaned forward to place myself within her grip. She squeezed me closer, placed her hand on the back of my head, right above my neck, and pulled me in. Our lips kissed, brief but meaningful.

"Hey sweetie," I replied.

Her eyelids opened slowly, and as she looked at me, she tilted her head a little to one side. One eyebrow raised higher than the other, as if she noticed something different.

"You okay honey?" she asked.

She must have spotted the remnants of my emotional breakdown earlier. I am sure the redness of my eyes had not completely disappeared yet, even though I vigorously splashed cold water on my face trying to clear any signs of crying. I cupped her face in my right hand, stroked my thumb along her cheekbone, soft and gentle.

"I am fine sweetie," I said.

She knew. She was aware of the little white lie, but accepted it as such and chose not to ask anything else.

Becky's mother was sitting in a chair close to the end of her bed. One hand resting on the mattress, as if she were trying to connect physically with Becky through it. She had that beautiful grey hair that only few people are blessed with. Her eyes normally radiated joy, but now, they were emitting sorrow. She was worried and she had all the reasons for that. It was difficult for me to hold back my suspicion, but I had to. I could not say anything since we still did not have any results back from the biopsy. I walked over to her, greeted her and gave her a kiss on the cheek.

As I started to walk back to the opposite side of the bed, Becky explained that she called her earlier to tell her about the hospital stay. I sat down on the bed, right next to Becky's feet, facing her. As our hands reached each other, our fingers intertwined. Becky's mother stood up and explained that she was going back home. She had been sitting most of the day in the hospital with Becky in these uncomfortable chairs. She told us that one of Becky's siblings made plans to come to town, and that she would be here tomorrow morning.

She walked over to Becky, gave her a hug and a kiss and said,
"I will be back tomorrow."

She walked around the bed and as she placed a hand on my shoulder, she asked,

"The boys are taken care of, right?"

I confirmed that Lisa was at our home. She nodded, smiled, and walked out the room.

Five

I was awake before the nurse would eventually burst into the room for the early morning hospital routine. Becky was laying on her favorite side, the right side, and sleeping peacefully. Her chest was expanding in a slow and equally paced pattern, then, after a little pause, it would gently decrease in size. Ever since they started her on frequent breathing treatments, her cough was much better under control than before. She would still have some coughing spells here or there, but it was so much better.

The room was dark, but my eyes were adjusted enough to see everything. Today would be a different day; the results of the biopsy should come in and we would finally have a definite diagnosis, no more guessing. Deep down I knew that this news was going to be horrific and disastrous. Nonetheless, I still had some hope for a different outcome. Anything less than cancer would be better. I stretched my arm out and gently laid my hand on Becky's bed, my fingers barely touching her back. Not waking her, just touching her. Normally our bodies would cuddle together every night. She would always fall asleep in my arms. I missed her soft skin, her smell, her warmth. Just touching her back with my fingers gave me a feeling of togetherness. She did not move; her breathing continued to be calm and peaceful.

Doctor Johnson was sitting on a chair right in front of us. His hands folded in his lap, as if he were praying. He was in his mid-40's, goatee, normal build. I remember that he once had a student with him in the

ER, and that he was training him how to place a chest tube. He was showing the student where to make the incision, how to advance the tube, and how to assure the suctioning was working properly. I remember that he was a great teacher; very calm, well spoken, and he was very kind to both the patient and the student.

Now here he was, sitting in front of us. His eyebrows somewhat frowned, his face grim. Becky and I were both sitting on the bed. Becky had her legs folded beneath her, sitting upright, holding my hand. I was on the edge of the bed with both my legs hanging off the side. My left hand holding on to hers, while my right hand was flat on the bed as if I were trying to keep myself upright. It felt like we were both sitting at the principal's office because we were in trouble.

He took a deep breath in, unfolded his hands from his lap, placed one on his left leg, while the other opened up to emphasize what he was going to say. I noticed a slight tremble in his voice. Although barely evident, it was there. He tried to suppress it.

"Well…," he started, "the results from the biopsy are back."

Another deep breath followed by a sigh, as if he was trying to find strength before moving on.

"Becky, as I told you yesterday, you are very, very sick."

A sudden collection of liquid appeared in the corner of his eye. His upper lip started to tremble as he pushed back his tears,

"You have stage IV, non-small-cell lung cancer."

Silence filled the room, devastatingly loud. Unable to avoid this painful muteness, I looked at Becky. She had a blank numb stare. Not willing to give in to this news she fired back,

"So, it is not pneumonia."

Doctor Johnson turned his head towards her and with his watery eyes he looked straight at her.

"Oh, I wish Becky," he exclaimed, "but all the tests we have done, along with the biopsy, have confirmed that it is lung cancer, and that it has spread throughout your body."

He continued to have a difficult time, still fighting his emotions. His voice cracked when he proceeded to explain that there was not much they could do besides chemotherapy and maybe try a clinical trial.

"I want you to cut it out of me ..." Becky said desperately.

She started to tap on her chest with her hand. Her eyes filled with despair, her voice frightful.

"I need you to cut it out of me, please."

Hearing her desperation and fear ripped my heart out of my chest. Her hand now squeezing mine, her other hand rested on her chest. Her eyes filled with misery, and tears fell silently. I could not fathom the horror she was going through at that moment. Even to me, it was still a shock. I still had some hope for better news than this. Now it was official, a death sentence, a slow execution.

His clarification of why surgery would not be an option was delightfully simple. He explained,

"When you have a dandelion and it releases its seeds, the seeds are attached to those little fuzzy balls, right?"

Becky confirmed understanding by nodding and a "mhmhm" sound.

"When you blow on the dandelion and all those fluffy balls take off, they will land somewhere in the yard," he continued to explain.

"Then everywhere a little fuzz-ball lands, a new dandelion will grow."

"Okay..." Becky said.

"Your body is the yard and the dandelion is the cancer. Even if we cut out the main dandelion from the yard, all the other seeds will still grow to be dandelions."

Becky lowered her eyes, gazing at the floor. Her hand never stopped squeezing mine, the skin around her knuckles turned white, her shoulders hanging. I knew her mind was still trying to grasp all this information and understand this devastating news.

I looked at her, placed my other hand on top of hers and trapped it between both my hands,

"We will fight this babe; I will be right here with you."

She looked up, her eyes locked onto mine, our souls connected, and without words she explained her trust in me. She knew I would not give in or give up. My commitment to her was rocksteady and solid. We both stood in a dark place with a horrific storm around us tearing our skin, ripping the flesh off our bodies, but as long as we had each other, we could have a chance to pull through this.

Doctor Johnson explained that because the diagnosis was cancer, Becky would have to see an oncologist before she could be discharged from the hospital. He would contact them this morning and have an oncologist stop by later that afternoon so that Becky could go home later that day.

Both her hands were in mine. We were still sitting on the bed. I looked her straight in the eyes. The devastation was roaming inside her. I knew she was lost. I had to provide guidance and offer hope.

"Listen," I started, "we will do whatever we can do to fight this."

Her eyes stared hopefully at me.

"Besides the conventional medical treatment, I think we should look at different, more holistic options," I said.

"Okay," she responded, "But I do not know how."

"I have already done some research, and there are many other options out there," I explained.

I told her about some of the different treatment plans out there, both conservative and progressive. She sat up in bed and seemed more hopeful. I knew she was scared, but hope is a powerful ally.

The floor nurse informed us that the oncologist was going to stop by later that afternoon, and that this person would complete the discharge paperwork so Becky could go home.

"I will go home and pick up the boys from Kids Club," I said.

"I will also have to tell them what is going on."

We knew that it was important to be honest with them. This was a task I did not look forward to, but I took that burden upon myself so Becky did not have to worry about that.

"I know that it is important for us to be open with the boys," I said, "we cannot keep this information from them. We have to be honest, although it is difficult."

She slowly nodded.

"You are right sweetie," she said, "it is important for them to know. Thank you for doing that."

I leaned forward and rested my forehead against hers. We both closed our eyes and for a moment, we were one, emotionally completely connected. She gently moved forward and kissed my lips.

"I love you," she whispered. Her voice revealed her unconditional love.

"I love you too, babe." I said.

Some family members were there with Becky as I left to get Connor and Dane from Kids Club. As I moseyed down the hallway with my head slanted forward, my eyes locked onto the floor. I was thinking about this morning and how to explain this to our boys. I heard the increasing speed of footsteps behind me. They were getting louder and faster, but I chose not to pay attention. Suddenly, a hand landed on my shoulder, followed with an almost immediate

"Roy..."

Although I recognized the voice, I could not immediately place it. I halted my body, straightened my back, and as I started to turn around, the owner of the hand and voice came alongside me to face me directly. Her hair short and grey, her eyes gentle, and her smile warm. Her hand was still resting on my shoulder as she exclaimed,

"I am so sorry to hear about what is going on with Becky."

It was the House Supervisor of the hospital. She would usually spend many nights in the ER, as most of the action would occur in our department. She was a kind person with a compassionate heart. She explained that she was informed about the diagnosis because it involved the spouse of an employee.

"We just want to make sure that you and Becky are well taken care of," she justified.

"I know that the Cancer Center of Iowa will be sending someone to do the initial consult later this afternoon," she explained.

After she told me that the oncologist on-call would have to discharge Becky, she revealed that her daughter was also recently diagnosed with cancer. She swallowed her tears,

"But I am not here to talk about my daughter, I am here to let you know that we are very pleased with Doctor Freeman from the cancer center."

She explained that we might want to request him this afternoon when the other oncologist would stop by. After I thanked her for her help, we hugged each other.

"I will stay in touch with you guys," she said.

"Okay," I said, smiling at her.

I decided to take the main entrance instead of the employee exit, I did not want to walk by all of my colleagues and get confronted with questions about how Becky was doing. I knew they all cared, but I was just not ready for the confrontation at that particular moment; not now, maybe later.

The large revolving door at the main entrance detected my approach and automatically started to turn. As I passed through the glass rotating corridor, I could feel the cool pleasant air pass by me as I stepped into a fiery bowl of steaming hot air. Instantly my clothes stuck to my skin and several beads of sweat appeared on my forehead. The walk to my truck in the employee parking lot was only a short five-minute leisurely stroll. I was racking my brain for options on how to tell the boys. I knew I had to be honest, even though that was going to be a difficult and painful task.

My truck was in sight, I pulled the keys from my pocket, found the remote, and activated the remote start. The headlights flashed twice and I could hear the engine. Getting the air-conditioning started from here would cool the truck down some by the time I got there.

As I drove off the employee parking lot, I dialed Lisa's number. I needed to talk to her about Becky's official diagnosis, and I needed to tell her that I would pick the boys up from Kids Club to give them the awful news.

"Stage IV, that's the final stage," she exclaimed. The silence on the phone revealed her sadness.

"I am not giving up, Lisa," I said.

I shared my information with her about my research of the Moerman therapy from the Netherlands and the other information I discovered during my investigation for treatment options.

Picking up the boys today was different. They acted as wild and energized as usual. It was my mind that kept wandering off. Trying to determine the best strategy to tell them the news.

Honesty is most important, I thought, but I still wanted it to be as painless as possible.

Lisa would be back at the house around five. If I left right after she arrived, I would be back at the hospital in time before the oncologist would arrive. That gave me about an hour with the boys. A long and difficult one, but it had to be done.

I was ransacking my feelings and my logical mind to use the right words, the right tone, the right approach. I am not sure if the boys even noticed my silence during the car ride home. They were probably just very happy to see me. Their regular routine was completely thrown off after Becky and I went to the hospital just a few days ago.

The cool air from inside the house welcomed us home. Connor and Dane busted through the front door, running up the stairs towards the living room, making enough noise to alert the whole neighborhood. They were both pumped up because it was the weekend and Mama would be coming home soon. I walked up the stairs and headed for the kitchen to make myself a cup of tea. The boys wanted to play on the X-box and as they were deciding which game to play, I interfered.

"Guys, you can play in a little while, but first take your backpacks to your room, and after that I have to talk to you both, ok?"

I lowered a tea-bag into an empty mug, added some honey, then slowly drowned it with steaming water. With my mug in my hand, I slowly walked back to the living room. The boys still in their rooms, they had gotten sidetracked by something they found there. Their voices were noticeable in the distance. My chair felt comfortable. I placed my mug on the table next to me as it was still way too hot to consume.

"Connor, Dane, come here guys, I need to talk to you for a little!"

My voice cracked, just enough to be noticeable, while calling them. My hands were clammy, my heartbeat strong and pounding in my throat. They rushed into the living room, rambling about some new game they wanted to have. I lifted the tea from the table, carefully blew over the hot surface, tried a small sip, and made a soft slurping sound. Still too hot for comfort. I placed the mug back on the table and continued to get the boys to sit down. Tapping my hand on the ottoman in front of me, signaling the boys where I would like them to take a seat. Both understood my gesture and landed right next to each other, facing me, on the ottoman.

My eyes looked straight ahead at them, but not focused. My mind was still twisting and turning, wondering how to tell them, and worrying about how they would react. Would they understand the severity of it all? Would they cry or be upset? I could feel the wave of uneasiness flowing through my body.

"Well," I started, "the good news is that mama is getting home later this afternoon."

Their faces lit up with big smiles. I continued before they could say anything.

"Lisa will be here in a little while so I can go pick Mama up from the hospital, ok?"

Both boys were excited as could be.

"Yay, Mama is coming home!" they both shouted.

Although difficult, I had to continue. I did not want to devastate their world, but there was no escape.

"But there is also something not so good I have to tell you…"

Gently their clamor turned to silence, as if someone turned down the volume knob on the stereo. Their eyes locked on me, waiting for what I had to say. I had no clue how to say it with their big eyes staring at me; piercing through me. I had no clue how to package it properly so it would hurt less. I knew there was no other way but to be honest and straight, so I just jumped into the deep end.

"Guys, Mama is very sick. She has lung cancer."

Connor's eyes sprung wide open, his lips fell apart, his skin tone suddenly pale, his gaze full of disaster and devastation. He knew how bad this was and he realized all too well the impact of this destructive news.

Dane's stare became blank, empty as if he were not there, as if he didn't hear these painful words. He was just sitting there, in shock, motionless, like a statue. How I wish we were not there, not in this room, not in this situation. But regardless, here we were. A hurricane of destruction around us, ripping apart our lives.

Connor was finally able to bring out some words. With tears in his eyes, he stuttered.

"But...but...people die from cancer."

Dane's silence was heartbreaking. He still wasn't responding. I knew it was going to be harsh to be this honest, but there was no easy way of telling this gently.

"Well, Connor, that is true, but there are also still a lot of people that survive cancer," I explained. Both Connor and Dane were hanging on my lips, absorbing all the information like little sponges.

"Mama and I still need to talk to all the doctors and see what kind of treatment they are planning to do."

I also explained to them that we would do anything within our capabilities to fight off this gruesome disease. I shared with them my recently discovered information during my research, and both boys seemed very interested in getting all the information I had. I also wanted to make sure they knew that they could always ask me anything.

"And whenever you have any questions guys, please come to me right away ok?"

I tapped both my hands, one on each side of me, on the leather seat,

"Come sit here with me," I told the boys.

They came over from the ottoman, crawled against me, Connor on the left, Dane on the right. I covered them with my arms, holding them tight to me, trying to protect them from harm. I kissed them on their little heads.

"No matter what boys, both Mama and I we will be here for you, ok?"

A soft "mhmh" from Dane.

A depressed "okay" from Connor.

I offered to play a game with them on the X-box, trying to get their minds off this painful news. They always enjoyed playing a game with me, especially when they could gang up against me. Of course, when they would win, the victory dances were adorable. Nothing else would provide me more joy and lift my spirit than to see their happy faces jumping up and down, hands in the air, big smiles, and loud exclamations of their amazing capabilities of defeating me. We still had some time left before Lisa would be here, so we decided to play some games until I had to go pick up Becky.

My plan seemed to work as they became very occupied with the game and it appeared as if nothing were wrong. A triple knock on the front door. I could hear the door handle screeching quietly as it was being pushed down, and the door was gradually being pushed inward.

"It's just me!" Lisa announced.

We met each other at the top of the stairs. Her eyes red and watery, she wrapped her arms around me, pulling me close. She was shivering.

"This is so unfair," she whispered in my ear.

"I know," I said.

We both tried to shake off the negativity and walked towards the living room where Connor and Dane were still sitting on the ottoman, staring at the TV and moving their fingers rapidly on the controllers.

"Hey guys!" Lisa threw their way to get their attention.

Both boys dropped their game controllers and jumped up, ran towards her as if they had not seen her for months. Lisa was welcomed by many hugs and kisses. They truly loved her.

Traffic was thick this late in the afternoon, especially because it was a Friday. The ride to the hospital was painstakingly slow. As usual at this time of the day, the number of visitors at the hospital was also at a peak, causing me to decide to take the stairs again. Becky's door was closed, so out of courtesy I knocked before placing my hand on the door handle and pushing it open. I stepped through the doorway and peeked around the door to stare right at Becky. Her eyes perked up and a big smile appeared,

"Hey babe," she said.

I stepped toward her, greeted the family that was sitting there, and as usual Becky raised her arms up to the sky to welcome me with a loving hug followed by a kiss that would only last a few seconds, but leave an imprint for a lifetime.

"How were the boys?" she asked.

She focused on every word I said, hanging on my lips as if her life was depending on it, her head tilting from one side to the other with frequent smiles coming from her lips. I knew she was missing her boys, and I knew that she wanted to spare them from the atrocious news about the cancer that was trapped inside her body. A sheen glazed over her eyes, a single tear escaped and rolled down her cheek where it was wiped away by her fingers.

My hand reached out to her face, the connection between my hand to her cheek caused her to tilt her head just enough to entrap it between her shoulder and her cheek. As she kissed the inside of my hand, her eyes looked up at me, and while I drowned in her gaze from her dazzling green emeralds, she proclaimed,

"I love you."

I told her about my meeting with the house supervisor in the hallway. How she vouched for the oncologist that was in charge of her daughter's treatment plan.

"Well, let's meet him first before we decide," Becky said.

As we were exchanging experiences from the day, a soft

"Hello?" came into the room, followed by,

"Are you Becky Slootheer?"

A female in her mid-50's with short gray hair and a business dress was standing in the door opening. She had a kind face, pleasant smile, and soft tone of voice. Becky confirmed. The lady stepped forward, holding out her hand toward Becky. With a short shake of the hands, she introduced herself as the oncologist from the cancer center. She would be completing the initial patient assessment.

She was one of the many oncologists that were part of a larger group known as the *Cancer Center of Iowa*. A binder was clamped under her left arm. She pulled up one of the chairs that was standing in the corner of the room. After placing the chair to face Becky, she sat down, positioned the binder on top of her legs, placed both her hands on it and looked straight at Becky. She conveyed a lot of information to the both of us, consistently shifting her attention between Becky and me.

We had a long conversation about the possible treatment plans. She also explained that it would be important to have some additional testing done on the biopsy sample. There was a possibility that the cancer was caused by a gene-mutation. If this were the case, the treatment plan would change completely. She would order this testing, but it would take several weeks before we would receive the results.

We made her aware that we would like to have a discussion with Doctor Freeman to determine if we would like to use him as our oncologist. She explained she would gladly contact his assistant to make an appointment for us next week.

The discharge process did not take long. Within 30 minutes after the oncologist left, the floor nurse arrived with all the necessary paperwork. Although it was a tedious process, with lots of signatures and initialing, it did not take much longer than 20 minutes. While Becky and I were going through the discharge papers with the nurse, the family members left. They told us that they would come to the house the following day.

Once we were done with all the discharge papers, the floor nurse was going to take Becky to the exit with a wheelchair.

"Why don't you go ahead and get the car. We will meet you downstairs," she told me.

"By the time you get the car and drive to the main entrance, we should be arriving at the main entrance."

I smiled to express my understanding. I leaned forward towards Becky, kissed her lips and said,

"Love you babe, see you in a bit."

"Ok sweetheart," while she smiled and looked at me with those bright green eyes.

The welcoming committee at home involved two young boys, that had been without their mama for way too long, and a great friend with a big heart that was ready to see her best friend back home. When I pushed the door handle and opened the front door, they knew it was us. The stampede of four little feet on the hardwood floor created a joyful moment for both Becky and me. We briefly looked at each other, smiled and shook our heads. We barely walked into the house, had not even set a foot on the stairs yet, and they came bursting down like a wave that was crashing onto the beach. Then they latched onto Becky's body and did not let go.

Finally, they allowed her to walk and we all proceeded up the stairs, us slowly, the boys like wild animals. At the top, Becky was greeted by Lisa, arms wide open, tears flowing over her cheeks, and a big smile.

"Oh Becky, I am so glad you are back home."

Her tears were a combination of joy because she was back home, and sadness from the cancer diagnosis. Lisa was not going to say anything. She was determined to be here for Becky.

Becky got to our chair and comfortably cuddled in the middle as both boys jumped on board to sit right next to her. I decided to leave them together and sit right next to Lisa on the love seat. Time flew by faster than expected. It was almost eleven when Lisa decided it was time for her to go home and get some much-needed sleep. We said goodbye to Lisa, and as she walked out the door she shouted,

"I love you all!"

Becky got the boys to bed and snuggled with them for some time. She back-stepped out of their rooms as they exchanged blowing kisses and 'I love you's'. It was a joy to see them all happy. It was amazing to have Becky back home. We both crawled in bed. After 13 years of marriage, we had created our own spots to sleep. She cupped my face with both her hands, slowly lowered her eyelids to a close, pulled me closer, kissed me with an unexplainable intensity, and said,

"Goodnight sweetheart. I love you!"

She positioned herself on her right side and curled up.

I moved closer to her, my right arm along her pillow and my left wrapped around her. My body against her, my face along her neck and back of her head, her skin soft and warm, her smell intoxicating. I closed my eyes and as I drowned in perfection, laying right next to her, I fell, deep, into darkness, numbness, silence...

Six

The morning came soft and tender. Sunlight breezed through the bedroom and caressed my face gently. I slowly raised my eyelids from a comfortable, deep, and well-deserved sleep. Becky's body warm along my side, her smell invigorating, her skin soft as silk. For a brief moment it felt as if I had awakened from a bad dream. A plastic bag from the hospital filled with clothing, still standing on the chair in the corner of our bedroom, destroyed that possibility.

A feeling of nervousness combined with nausea presented itself again inside my stomach. I glared over at my alarm-clock, standing lonely on a wooden pedestal, telling me it was 7:15am. Becky was still sound asleep. I am sure she was glad to be back in her own bed again.

I snuck from underneath the comforter as sly as possible, like a cat gliding through the grass approaching his prey. I tried not to disturb anything in the bed, so Becky could continue with her much-needed rest. Successfully I completed my silent moves and stood beside the bed. With a triumphant feeling of victory, since Becky was still sleeping undisturbed, I tip-toed through the bedroom towards the hall. My eyes never lost contact of her, just to make sure I did not wake her.

In the hallway I continued my light treading, almost floating. I walked past the boys' room and peeked inside. They were both still in dreamland. I continued my path towards the kitchen. On my way to the dining room table I passed the coffee maker. A simple flip of the switch started the brewing process. I had set it up the night before to get it going easily in the morning. While the machine started to make soft sputtering noises, I took my place at the dining room table. I was facing the hallway just in case Becky or the boys came out of bed, so I would see them right away. I opened my laptop and automatically it came to life.

My coffee cup, filled with steaming black goodness, was standing guard right next to my laptop. I turned my cell phone to silent and placed it right below my coffee, keeping it within eyesight just in case someone needed to get a hold of me. The notepad and pen were awaiting my orders for the recording of vital intelligence. I was ready to continue my quest for knowledge and information.

My fingers danced perfectly choreographed over the keyboard. The screen presented a magnitude of information about fighting cancer with juicing, the Moerman's diet, the Gerson therapy, Vitamin C infusions in Mexico, and hyperthermia treatments in Germany. An overflow of information continued to pour over the monitor. My brain analyzed the material, separating the important data from the worthless.

I continued to jot down website addresses, data, telephone numbers and other material I wanted to look into later. Several cups of coffee passed by when suddenly my phone made a soft buzzing sound. It caught me by surprise, and I jumped as if something just bit me. I jerked my head to the right and observed the screen. It was a text message from Becky,

'Where you at?'

I gently pushed the chair backwards and stood up. I realized that I had been sitting at the table for almost three hours.

"I am right here babe," I said, as I started to walk down the hallway towards our bedroom.

"I just woke up," Becky said, "and I didn't hear anything. I was not sure where you were at."

I explained that I was trying to be quiet, and it seemed I did a good job because everyone was still asleep.

"Let me make you some breakfast babe," I said, "I am sure the boys would want some scrambled eggs and pancakes too."

She gladly accepted that offer. She always proclaimed that I made the best scrambled eggs on the planet; not too dry, not too moist, just perfect.

Everyone was sitting at the dining room table as I served the early morning meal. The boys gobbled up their eggs and pancakes as if they had not been fed for days. Becky, on the other hand, had a couple of bites, then told me that her stomach was just not feeling well. After she explained that she was still very tired, she said that she wanted to go back to bed and rest for a little.

She stood up very slowly. I noticed that she was weak. As I helped her stand, I wrapped my right arm around her, and placed my left hand in front of her for her to hold on to. She grabbed it for support, tilted her head to the left, looked straight into my eyes, and smiled.

"I am sorry sweetie, but I guess I am just still really tired."

I smiled back, kissed her softly on her lips and responded,

"No worries babe. It is ok."

We shuffled together through the kitchen into the hallway like an old couple in their late 80's.

As I got Becky to bed, right before she curled up on her side, she reached over and grabbed my hand. She looked at me with soft moist eyes. I could feel her soul inside shiver, afraid, and scared.

"I am sorry babe," she said softly.

But these words were delivered with such intensity and feeling, I could sense her pain and fear. Without letting go of her hand, I sat down on the edge of the bed, right next to her. She curled her body like a fetus around me, her shoulder making small erratic movements as tears streamed over her face. Through her pain with short bursts of inhalation she confessed, her voice quivering and filled with despair,

"I am so scared babe."

I leaned forward, covering her body with mine, like a blanket trying to comfort and protect her. My hand not letting go of hers, with the other hand, I ran my fingers slowly through her hair. I whispered in her ear,

"We will find a way, sweetheart, don't give up."

Her body was now in full shuddering mode, her eyes closed, tears falling rapidly. Her hand squeezed mine, her fingers entrapped mine so hard that her knuckles turned white.

I have to stay strong. I have to be her rock. I must find a solution.

I kept thinking these words while I continued to comfort her. As minutes slipped by, Becky's breathing became deep and relaxed; she was falling asleep. I just sat there with her for a moment, holding her hand, watching her.

My soul reached out to her, trying to give her strength. I could not fathom what she was going through. How scary this must be for her. I closed my eyes,

'Dear God, please, please help my sweet Becky. Please help her heal and beat this horrible cancer. If there is someone that can make this happen, it is You. Please God, please.'

Tears fell along my cheeks and with a quick swipe from my hand, they were removed. I could hear the boys playing a game in the living room. I gradually removed myself from the bed. Becky did not respond, her breathing stayed constant. I pulled the comforter up over her shoulder, went into the hallway, softly moving towards the living room. Connor and Dane were hypnotized staring at the game on the TV. Before I sat down behind them, I kissed their little faces, and reminded them,

"Guys, mama is asleep, so keep it quiet, ok?"

Both of them, almost synchronized, replied, "Ok Papa!"

I leaned back into my oversized chair and placed my legs on the ottoman behind the boys. The game that the boys were playing provided for a comforting mind-numbing experience. Suddenly the sound of my phone impolitely disturbed my detachment from the world. I brought the phone to my ear,

"Hello?".

It was one of the family members that wanted to stop by. I explained that Becky had just gone to bed and that she was sound asleep at that moment.

"Let me call you as soon as she wakes up, okay?" I said.

"Okay, that sounds like a plan," she responded.

***

Becky was sitting upright in bed, pale, hunched forward, holding a bucket, her shoulders making jerky movements as she was dry heaving. Some family members surrounded her, swarming around her like bees on a honey pot. I tried to imagine how difficult it had to be for them to see Becky this sick. I knew how it felt for me, to see the love of my life battling one of the most feared diseases on the planet. I tried to imagine the emotional whirlwind they were going through.

The fact that they were crowding Becky was not good, but understandable because all they wanted to do was to help her. Emotional stress can sometimes be the reason we lose our clarity of what is best. There was no question in my mind about their love and concern for Becky, but sometimes it is better to give a person some space, especially when a person is actively vomiting.

Suddenly someone started to force anti-nausea medicine to Becky. At that moment I knew for sure that clear judgement was lost. Giving someone anything by mouth that is actively vomiting is counterproductive. The moment it was going down, it would come back up almost instantly. Even if that medicine was supposed to make them feel better.

I tried to make clear to not give Becky anything orally for now, because she would throw it right back up. I assumed that person would understand but instead, it aggravated the situation and this person rebutted me. I was observing a family that was frustrated and struggling with intense emotional pain. That combined with the feeling of powerlessness and fear caused an unexpected attack towards me, and without making any sound, a four-letter-word was thrown my way.

It was my first exposure to awkward behavior from a family member. I raised my eyebrows, shocked from the message I had just received. Full of disbelief. It felt like someone just kicked me straight in the stomach. I was not mad, just hurt. An unexpected pain. This was an experience I had not anticipated; not now, not from a family member, not in this situation.

Up until now, I was convinced that we were all on the same team and had the same goals. It seemed though, that some were unable to maintain courtesy amongst those that care the most and were unable to understand that it was no one's fault; that we were all unwillingly thrown into this horrible event. Pointing fingers at each other would not make this situation any better.

People under stress make sudden and unpredictable moves. I understand that, but I did not foresee it happening here. I thought we were a tight group, with strong relationships, maybe that's why that moment was so painful.

Regardless of the attack, I decided to wave it off, blaming it on stress, and I took the high road. I walked out of the room without saying anything and went into the kitchen. I needed something to do just to get my mind off of the situation, a little break. I noticed some dirty dishes inside the sink and decided that cleaning them would be my mission for a while.

I hand-washed each plate, cup, and glass with immaculate precision. The situation in my bedroom seemed to calm down. Shortly thereafter, the individual came up to me and apologized.

"Sorry Roy, I should not have said that. I am really sorry. I am just under a lot of stress right now."

I accepted the apology and let it go. I understood that everyone deals with stress differently. Some become quiet, some cry, some laugh, others have to blame someone for the situation they are in.

The boys were in the big chair Becky and I always sat in. They wanted me to come sit with them while they were watching TV. Before I planted myself between them, I wanted to check on Becky to make sure she was doing well.

"I will be right back boys, just going to check on mama really quick."

With my cat-like stealth, I moved through the hallway. As I arrived at our bedroom, I peeked around the corner and saw that Becky sound asleep. I backed away silently.

"Mama is asleep," I announced while I lowered myself into the soft leather cushions.

I leaned back, both boys leaning with me, gazing at nothing interesting on TV, yet it provided some mental peace.

Ever since we got home, Becky struggled with fatigue. She could walk from the bed to the living room and back, but besides that, there was not much physical activity. She slept a lot throughout the day. I was sure that the cancer was eating away her energy, but also the pain medicine she was taking made her drowsy. Her nausea was probably caused by all the different medicines she was taking. I did let her sleep as much as possible, I figured she needed it. Her cough was much better controlled after we started doing frequent breathing treatments at home.

Every morning I would wake up early to do my research, and today was no different. The sun had just started to break through the horizon. Becky was still asleep and both boys were also still snoozing away. Time for me to continue my research. Tomorrow we were scheduled to meet with Doctor Freeman, the oncologist, for the first time. So, today I wanted to focus on additional data from different treatment approaches.

Armed with my laptop, coffee, phone, notebook and a pen, I settled down at the dining room table. Many research results appeared on my screen, but the collective idea from most sources appeared to be nutrition; healthy, organic, non-genetically-modified-organism (GMO), non-dairy, a minimum of meats, fish, and poultry. Juicing of vegetables and fruits also played an important role in natural healing. The closer to the vine, the better the nutritional value for healing and repair of the cellular structure.

It was time for me to talk with a real-life person, so I decided to call 'The Moerman Association' in the Netherlands. I knew it was seven hours later there, so I had to call early in the morning, before they closed for the day. Clinging on to my coffee with one hand, I opened the sliding door that led to our deck on the backside of the house. I tried not to make a sound, so I pushed slowly to minimize the friction that habitually caused a screeching noise that would curl up your skin and give you goosebumps, like someone scratching their fingernails on a blackboard.

I need to spray this thing with some WD-40, I thought while pushing the door open at an agonizing slow pace. The air outside was still comfortable from the cool night that just made way for the sun. I spotted dew drops on the grass delicately trailing down. The fresh early morning air tingled my senses. I closed my eyes and inhaled deeply, holding it for a split moment, and letting it go with a soft humming sound.

I placed my coffee cup on the ledge of the railing that surrounded the deck, pressed numbers on my phone and called the Netherlands. Within three rings, a young lady answered, her voice soft and kind, greeting me in Dutch. I explained to her about Becky's diagnosis, and that I was in search of additional information about the Moerman diet. She sounded very concerned and interested in Becky's situation as well as her treatment plan. She promised to send me information about the Moerman diet by email. More importantly, she gave me the personal phone number of one of the Dutch doctors who was very active in advising this diet to his cancer patients. After we ended our conversation, I immediately called this doctor. There was no answer, so I left him a detailed message and asked him to give me a call back.

Cautiously I moved the sliding door back open, stepped inside the house and slowly closed it again. I walked over to the counter where the coffee pot contained plenty of black juice to last me all morning. As I poured myself another cup of hot goodness, I heard a faint sound coming from the hallway. I leaned over to peek into the corridor that led to all of our bedrooms, but I did not see anything. I walked past the boys' rooms and both were still sleeping. The last room was our bedroom. As I moved closer, a sudden

"Honey?" greeted me from our room.

Becky was sitting upright in bed, smiling. We kissed.

"Morning babe," she said.

I sat down and told her about my morning, the research I had completed so far, my phone calls to the Netherlands, and all the information I'd discovered.

She tilted her head a little to the right, kept eye contact, and smiled.

"What?" I asked her.

"I could not have wished for a better husband," she said.

It was my duty, my mission to make sure she would get better. I would not let her down, nor would I deviate from that path. We talked for a long time about the different options, treatment plans, and changes we would have to make. Our decision was to use everything to our benefit to get the cancer under control; not only using conventional medicine, but also to change our diet to all natural and organic foods, to use certain supplements, and to start juicing fruits and vegetables.

The oncology clinic was conveniently located right next to the hospital, with its own entrance and valet parking service. The valet service consisted of two sweet old retired guys that took care of those in need. The waiting room was as any other; neutral appearance, uncomfortable chairs that you don't want to sit in too long, magazines on the table, and plastic plants randomly dispersed throughout the area. I never expected to sit at an oncology clinic, not even in my wildest dreams. Becky was sitting right next to me, holding my hand, not saying much, not knowing what to expect. Less than a week ago none of this was on our schedule. Now, we were sitting here, with our minds still blown, mentally numbed.

The day before our first oncology visit was my birthday. Three days after we got home from the hospital, three days after we received the mortifying news. There was nothing to celebrate, and I told Becky I did not want to have a birthday party, but she was very adamant in her approach and wanted to have some type of get together with family. She ordered a cake and we all went to her mother's house for cake and ice cream. I did not want to go but thought maybe it was better to do so. It would keep some normalcy and that was most important for the boys.

I remember we were all sitting at the long table, cake and ice cream on individual plates. Becky sitting next to me holding my hand, everyone singing,

"Happy birthday to you, happy birthday to you, happy birthday dear Roy..."

At that moment, I wanted to sink into the ground and fade away. I did not want to be there. My heart was heavy, my eyes filled with tears of pain and sorrow, my body numb. I forced a smile on my face to keep appearances, but inside I was crying and screaming.

'Happy birthday?' I was thinking, 'Happy?'

We just received the most bloodcurdling news, but they were singing 'Happy Birthday.' Nothing could be further from the truth.

The boys sang louder than ever, Becky smiled and sang at the top of her lungs, but in her eyes, I could see the pain and fear of the unknown. She was unable to hide it from me. She knew that I could see through her wall, and as her hand was holding mine, the gentle rubbing of her finger on the back of my hand explained more than words ever could.

A young lady appeared from the hallway that was hidden on the far-right side of the clinic, next to the check-in area. She called Becky's name, and we both stood up and walked over to her without letting go of each other.

"Hi," she said, "my name is Angie." She reached out her hand to shake ours.

"I am Doctor Freeman's nurse, please follow me."

Becky and I continued to hold hands while we followed her into the hallway, took a 90 degree turn to the right and then went into a room on the left. A desk along the wall with an office chair and a laptop. Two chairs and an exam table were placed on the opposite side.

Becky and I sat down right next to each other in the two chairs. Angie started to unravel the blood-pressure cuff, and while she was taking Becky's vital signs, she asked many questions about Becky's health and the medications she was taking. When she was finished, she told us that Doctor Freeman would be there soon, then left the room.

There was a soft knock. The door handle made a soft gentle clicking sound, then it was pulled open. A tall young man stepped into the room. He was in his mid-30s, friendly face, short brown hair, sparkly eyes, and a gentle smile. As he walked into the room, he reached his hand out towards Becky and announced,

"I am Doctor Freeman; you must be Becky?"

While she was shaking his hand, Becky confirmed his question. I was next. He placed his hand in mine and with a nice firm grip he gave it a couple of shakes and introduced himself. He told us to sit down while he lowered himself into the desk chair.

He was a very pleasant man, with a kind voice, soft and well spoken, calm, and with caring eyes. Although he was working in a field where death was no stranger, he had a positive yet realistic attitude. He was like a good friend that would put an arm around you when you needed to cry, but also speak the harsh truth if warranted. He allotted plenty of time for this meeting to allow us to ask any questions we had. His bedside manner was phenomenal, and I understood why the house supervisor of the hospital recommended him.

A lot of time was spent discussing the actual diagnosis of stage IV non-small-cell lung cancer, the impacts it would have, what to expect, and possible treatment plans. It was clear that Becky's situation was horrible; her future was grim. He explained that normally he would start chemotherapy but clarified that he wanted to wait with this aggressive plan because it has such a destructive effect on the human body.

"More frequently, many lung cancer patients with no clear cause for the disease can have a certain gene mutation that is the actual cause," he said.

"Okay …?" Becky responded, with her head tilted slightly to the right.

"If this would be the case, chemotherapy would not be the best initial treatment," he continued to explain.

"For certain gene mutations there is now a *targeted* medication available that can actually control the gene that is changing and causing the cancer."

"Oh," Becky said, "that's what the other doctor was explaining to us, right?" as she looked at me and nodded her head.

"Correct," Doctor Freeman said, "we can wait with the chemotherapy for a couple of weeks until we know for sure it is not caused by a gene mutation."

He continued to explain that we would also have to do a new biopsy since the previous biopsy did not allow for enough sample tissue to complete this specialized test. He also recommended Becky to get a port placed for easy access for medication administration and blood draws.

At some point during our conversation with him, he asked if we wanted to know the statistics for survival for this type of cancer. Without hesitation, both Becky and I, almost synchronized, responded with a clear

"NO!"

Even though Becky and I never discussed this, we were both on the same wavelength. We knew that the statistics were not good. We knew that most people that are diagnosed with this type of cancer do not make it past five years, some don't even make it past the first six months. Realistically, we did not care about those numbers because it was our plan to beat this horrible disease and Becky would be one of those miracle cases that survived.

On our way home, Becky grabbed my hand, her fingers entangling mine like an octopus entrapping its prey. I looked at her, her mouth small, pressed lips, her eyes showed concern and hope simultaneously.

"This is good right?" she asked.

The tone of her voice, the look in her eyes, and her body language told me how scared she was; she was terrified. I pulled the truck over to a parking lot. This was too important not to discuss. We needed to talk about this right away. She needed it, she deserved this time for just us to relay, discuss, and evaluate what was going on. No doctors, nurses, family members, or friends to interfere, just the two of us. I started to turn the wheel and aimed for a large parking lot along the street.

"What are you doing babe?" she asked.

"Let's talk for a second," I responded.

Her silence implied her approval. I parked the truck on an almost deserted parking lot. I unbuckled my seat belt and shifted my body to my right, so I was facing her. I cupped her hand with both my hands. Becky also turned her body to face me more directly. She was longing for my words, hanging on my lips, like a life-sustaining nectar she desired to digest for survival. She needed guidance and support: The comfort of knowing that not all was lost, that there still was hope.

"This is good news sweetheart," as I confirmed her previous remark.

"It is a good decision to see if this can be treated with oral medication first, instead of chemotherapy."

Becky smiled, her appearance blossomed up, the clouds seem to dissipate as my words injected hope and comfort into her veins.

"And that combined with the changes we are going to make, we are fighting this from all possible sides," I continued.

She moved forward, folded her arms around me, placed her body against mine, an enjoyable entrapment. She kissed my lips, moved her head along my cheek to rest it on the side of my face, and whispered,

"I love you. I cannot do this without you," and with that, our commitment was sealed, a partnership for life that I willingly accepted.

When we pulled up to the house, I saw Lisa's car on the driveway. We walked inside the house and there was an awkward silence. No greeting ceremony from the boys, no one standing at the top of the stairs, only stillness; nothing but lifeless air. Both of us climbed up the stairs to find an empty house without a living soul around. When we browsed through the kitchen, I noticed Lisa sitting on our deck, reading a book. Both boys were playing in our backyard. The large oak trees in the backyard created a comfortable shade that provided for some extra cooling. When I opened the sliding door, Lisa looked up, closed her book, placed it onto the table next to her and, as Becky and I walked onto the deck, she welcomed us with a big smile and a hug.

"Hey guys," she exclaimed enthusiastically.

Becky sat down next to Lisa and started to narrate everything about our meeting that morning with Doctor Freeman. Lisa just smiled, happy just to be there. The boys both came running onto the deck, each with a chicken in their arms, showing them to Becky as if they were trophies they'd won during a game.

We had purchased chickens about three months ago. We let them grow and kept them for their eggs. They would roam free on our land during the day, and at night they would go into their coop in the barn that was located in the back part of our land. It was amazing to see that they never left our property.

***

Becky got pregnant with Connor in December 1999, eight months after we got married. It was then that we decided it was time for us to move out of our townhouse. We needed something with more space and more rooms. Even though the townhouse had two bedrooms and could easily house a family with one child, we were ready to move. After we started looking around, we realized quickly that we both wanted to move to an area outside the city limits so we could have some additional land.

Within months of searching we found a great location, barely outside the city limits of a small local town, a four-bedroom split level on 5 acres. It was perfectly positioned on top of a hill, about five minutes away from everything a small family needed; the grocery store, medical facilities, and schools. Besides the location, both Becky and I wanted to have some extra land. We always talked about building a log-cabin style home, and this acreage would allow for that dream to come true.

After we moved in, during the first week of June 2000, we both roamed our property and decided where we would build our dream home; on top of a little hill on the south side of our property. It was surrounded by large oak trees and it would be facing nothing but woods and land. Perfect.

***

We sat on the deck for almost one hour, just talking away, when suddenly the air started to become thick and soggy. The humidity was increasingly sticking to our skin, suffocating it slowly with warm sultry, vicious moist air. Becky stood up, and although she normally enjoyed the heat, she made gestures that she was going inside where the temperature was more pleasant. I called the boys for them to come in and get something to drink. Becky and Lisa walked into the living room, as I started to make some fresh pressed apple juice for everyone.

The day before I bought a juicer so we could get started on the juicing program. Since the boys liked apple juice, I decided to start juicing all fruits at home instead of buying it processed. They actually liked it much better than the apple juice we usually bought in bottles.

The boys were sitting at the dining room table, discussing how to build a fort in the backyard, while gulping down the golden nectar I had just made for them. As I started to walk from the kitchen to the living room with two more glasses of nature's goodness, one for Becky and one for Lisa, the front door opened, and some family members walked in.

"Hey guys," I said, while I raised both my eyebrows at the same time as if I were using them to wave at them.

"We are all up here," inviting them to come up the stairs and join us.

Seven

Becky was sitting in her usual spot in our chair, and as always, I sat right next to her. Some family members and friends were visiting us. All of them scattered throughout the living room. The boys decided to take off and play outside, they didn't want to hang out with all the adults. Becky was talking to Lisa when suddenly my phone rang. I glanced at the screen to see who was calling, and if it was important enough for me to answer the call. It was an international number, from the Netherlands.

"Gotta take this babe," I told Becky.

"I think this is that Dutch doctor calling me back."

As I walked out of the room and onto the deck, away from all the noise, I answered the call,

"This is Roy."

A male voice on the other side responded in English with a thick Dutch accent. He introduced himself as the physician from the Moerman association that I had called a couple of days ago. I changed my language to Dutch. Although I had lived in the United States for over fifteen years, I still spoke my native language fluently.

After I explained Becky's diagnosis of stage IV non-small cell lung cancer, he told me that he started to advise his patients, that were struggling with cancer, to start following the Moerman diet. He was very impressed with the positive results for his own patients. He shared a lot of information with me, answered all my questions, and provided a better insight into the actual program. Our conversation lasted just short of an hour. He promised to send me additional material via email, including a diet guideline for Becky to follow.

I proudly delivered my newly discovered knowledge to Becky, our friends and family. Now we had detailed information about the Moerman diet. It was important for the family to know about this diet, so they would also be aware of what was included and what should be avoided. It was important that we were all on the same page.

One of Becky's sisters told us that she had been in contact with Doctor Crawford from the Duke Cancer Institute in Durham, North Carolina. Apparently, he is one of the leading oncologists that specifically deals with lung cancer. She explained that she had been talking with him, and that he was more than willing to see Becky and provide a second opinion. Getting a second opinion, especially if this oncologist is recognized as one of the leading experts in their field, is always a smart decision.

***

The sound of the engines was getting louder, the vibration gradually increasing, my seat was shaking. The force was being held back, until a certain limit was reached. Then, right before the pitch of the turbines seemed to indicate they would break down, all the energy was released. The disengagement of the constraining devices caused the silver bird to accelerate at an intense, rapidly developing speed.

I was being pushed back into my seat, my body pulsating on the rhythm of the power plants that were providing the thrust for this craft to be released from its containment on earth. The concrete runway passed the small oval window at an increasing pace until it actually defied gravity and detached itself from the ground to accelerate through the air at unimaginable heights. Its ability to take off and fly was both nerve-wracking and exciting at the same time.

Becky's hand was holding mine, our fingers intertwined, her knuckles turning white. She was staring straight ahead, breathing shallow and silent. She had never been afraid of flying, but earlier this year, in March, we had a horrible flight from Dallas to Fort Meyers. We had to fly between thunderstorms causing the plane to bounce up and down, left and right, with intense forces. It was a terrifying experience. That was five months ago, and this flight was much smoother.

Once we reached the planned cruising altitude and the engines slowed down, the flight attendants started to move around. The air was smooth, and Becky regained her comfort level. We had one stop in Minneapolis before arriving in Raleigh, North Carolina. We would be staying at the Washington Duke Inn. It was close to the cancer institute where we had an appointment with Doctor Crawford for the following day.

A large open atrium welcomed us to the facility. A friendly lady with a heavy southern accent at the information desk provided us with clear directions on how to get to Doctor Crawford's clinic on the second level. Becky and I discussed our plan for a second opinion with Doctor Freeman prior to arriving here. He actually promoted the idea to go and meet with Doctor Crawford. All of Becky's medical files was going to be send to his office, so Doctor Crawford could review them before our arrival here today.

Just a couple of minutes after we were brought to the exam room, the door opened and a gentleman with dark blond hair, parted in one direction, and a short stubby goatee, walked into the room. His presence filled the room with compassion and kindness. He stretched out his hand towards Becky,

"You must be Becky," he said. "It is so nice to meet you. I am Doctor Crawford."

They connected hands and as they shook, he placed his left hand on top of Becky's hand.

"Nice to meet you," Becky replied.

After his introduction to Becky, he turned towards me, reached out his hand, and as I connected with him, he confirmed,

"You then must be Roy, very nice to meet you."

His grip was comfortably firm.

After he conducted some physical assessments, he sat down on the rolling stool and moved closer towards Becky.

"Becky," he started with a serious and concerning tone in his voice,

"I reviewed your file that was sent to me by Doctor Freeman, and I looked at all the images and the results from all the tests."

Becky reached for my hand, and as she got a hold of it, she pulled me closer and placed both our hands together in her lap.

"I believe that Doctor Freeman has the right approach," he said, "The most important issue right now is to obtain another biopsy so we can determine if there is a gene-mutation."

He continued to look at us both as he explained.

"Until then, we should, as Doctor Freeman also recommended, wait."

Becky and I remained silent, our hands together, our souls connected.

We discussed many aspects of the diagnosis, treatment plan, and our decision to follow certain holistic steps. He endorsed every aspect we discussed. Doctor Crawford also carefully indicated that there could be some opportunities for clinical trials if all other options were exhausted. He promised that he would stay in contact with Doctor Freeman and on top of Becky's treatment plan.

"You can always contact me if you have any questions or concerns," he offered.

Before he left, he asked Becky if she would like to talk to one of the mental health care specialists from his clinic. Initially Becky hesitated, but Crawford was persistent about it.

"It is part of the whole treatment plan," he said. "I really would like you to talk to him for a little."

Becky hesitantly nodded and agreed to meet with him.

He was a young man in his mid-thirties. Dressed in business casual attire, sitting on the same stool Doctor Crawford was sitting on earlier. Becky moved from the exam table to one of the more comfortable chairs that were placed along the wall. As he started to explain about the psyche of the human mind, the emotional tidal waves a person will go through while dealing with a disastrous disease like this one, it was a painful relief to see that Becky actually started to talk. Maybe it was because he was not close to her heart, after all he was a complete stranger, and sometimes it is easier to pour your heart out to a person you don't know. Or maybe it was because it was just the right time and the right place.

She continued to hold my hand, not letting go, assuring her connection with me. Her voice became shaky, there were short moments of silence when she pushed back the tears. When he asked her about fears, she was unable to hold back her despair, her walls of protection started to tumble down, brick by brick. A stream of tears started to flow from her eyes, over her cheeks, landing silently in her lap. Her shoulders softly shaking, her body moving closer to mine. She placed her body against mine, seeking warmth, seeking compassion, seeking love. I wrapped my arm around her, pulling her closer. Her face rested in the corner of my neck, her hand not letting go of the grasp she had on mine.

My lips gently touched her forehead, and I softly whispered,

"It's ok sweetie, it's ok."

But on the inside, I was trembling. I was holding back my own tears, trying to stay strong for her. We were comfortably rocking back and forth as one unit. My eyes aimed at her, my thumb stroking her cheek and softly wiping away the tears of pain. My heart broke into a thousand little pieces seeing her in so much agony, so much fear, so scared, terrified for what was coming her way; ruthless and inevitable. We just sat there, minutes passed by, just her and I, silently together.

The counselor contained his words. He knew not to speak at this moment, he knew this was needed and his expertise was proven by his silence.

The rubber of the wheels made a soft high-pitched noise as they came in contact with the concrete runway. The loud sound from the engines indicated that they were being used for break-assistance. The rapid deceleration caused a forward pull on our bodies, the seat belt tightening around my waist. The uneventful flight back was smooth and without any delays. The blistering heat outside caused a subtle distortion of the air rising up from the runway, disfiguring the view of the airport.

Like a newly married couple, we walked hand in hand through the terminal towards the baggage claim to collect the single suitcase we packed for this short trip. My truck was conveniently parked in the parking garage just across the airport. The air-conditioned walkway to the parking lot allowed us to avoid the sweltering heat outside. It was about three in the afternoon, which meant it was the hottest time of the day.

My left hand was holding on to the suitcase handle, rolling beside me. My other hand was holding on to Becky's. I parked the suitcase just behind the truck, unlocked the doors and walked in front of Becky to open the door for her. While I stood there, holding her door, she came close, kissed me, and stepped into the truck. I gently closed her door and walked towards the back to place the suitcase inside the truck-bed.

The next day Becky would get her port placed, and at the same time they would do a biopsy of the supraclavicular lymph node. They wanted to do it all in one sitting, just to make it easier for Becky. It would be an outpatient procedure and Becky was scheduled early in the morning. It would still take several weeks, after the biopsy was sent to the lab, to get the actual results.

Doctor Freeman made it clear that it would be very beneficial if there was a mutation because it would give more treatment options in the long run. If there was no gene mutation, the only option for treatment would be chemotherapy. Besides the devastating side effects, it would control the cancer for a while, but eventually it would find a way around it and continue to grow. If there was a gene mutation, the initial therapy would be oral medication that would target the gene causing the cancer. Then, if that failed there would still be the option for chemotherapy.

The OR nurse came through the sliding doors. She walked towards me and asked me to follow her. While we were walking to the recovery area, she told me that Becky had just arrived back from the OR and, although she was still falling in and out of anesthesia, she allowed me to come back and sit with her.

I placed a chair right next to her bed. She was sleeping. Beige hospital blankets covered her body, but both her arms were laying on top of the blankets. She was wearing the 'stylish' blue hospital gown. On her right wrist there was a white hospital bracelet with her information on it, and a half full IV bag hanging from the metal pole, dripping fluids into her system. My hand slid into hers, my fingers on the inside of her wrist, my thumb entrapping her hand, she did not move. My mind started to drift while I was sitting there, to memories not that long ago.

She was wearing the same gown, it was the same hospital, only several floors above us. The mother-baby floor. Becky was ready to give birth to our first child. She started to have more frequent contractions throughout the day, so she called the OB-GYN that evening. He instructed us to pack a bag and start heading towards the hospital. We got to the floor around 10pm. After some tests were completed, they determined that if nothing happened before midnight, they would start with medication to speed things up. Becky was determined to deliver our child naturally, without an epidural.

Midnight came and not much had transpired. They used Pitocin to trigger activity and the nurse explained that it could still take hours before anything would happen. Since Becky and I already had a long night, we decided to get some sleep. Becky curled up in her bed, I grabbed a pillow and some blankets to get some sleep on the couch that was located at the other end of the room. I think it only took me two minutes to fall into a complete coma.

The Pitocin worked way faster than expected. Becky's water broke within twenty minutes, and the moment she realized what happened, she tried to wake me up by calling my name. When I did not respond to her calls, she started to increase the volume of her voice several times, but without success. She decided to throw things at me to get my attention. I am glad that she had plenty of pillows because she explained that it took about 3 of them before she hit me right on the head and woke me up. I wonder what she would have thrown at me after she ran out of pillows?

Dazed and confused, I sat straight up and Becky softly yelled,

"Roy! Get over here! My water broke!"

As the night progressed, her pain came to a point that was unbearable for her. The moment she was completely silent, and stared straight ahead, I knew the misery was getting too much.

The nurse asked if she wanted something for pain, Becky squeezed my hand, looked at me and just nodded. The epidural was ordered and placed within thirty minutes. Six hours later we had a beautiful baby boy, healthy, and screaming at the top of his lungs.

Now Becky was in the same hospital, in the same gown, but not dealing with happy news. Instead, she was dealing with this disastrous, horrible disease that kills so many every year. I felt a sudden soft squeeze in my hand. I looked up into two bright green emeralds accompanied by a beautiful smile. I raised myself up from the chair, placed my hand on the bed for support, and welcomed her back with a gentle kiss.

"Hey babe, how are you feeling?" I asked.

"Doing well," she said, still somewhat drowsy.

***

School had started earlier that week. Both boys were actually happy to go back to school, but sad at the same time because the summer break was over. Since Becky still struggled a lot with the lack of energy, I brought them to school every morning, and picked them up every afternoon. Becky tried to come along as much as she could, but today was not a good day. She had not been feeling well since the moment she woke up. Intermittent episodes of dizziness and nausea, and no appetite. When it was time for me to pick up the boys, I told her,

"I will be right back baby," delivered a quick kiss, and left.

The school was only ten minutes away from our home, but since Connor was going to Junior High, and Dane to the Sixth-Grade center, they were in separate buildings. Because of that, their schools ended at different times, ten minutes apart. It would take me about thirty minutes to get back home. As usual I parked my truck in the middle of the parking lot that was conveniently located between the Junior High and the Sixth-Grade center.

I was standing in front of the four large doors of Connor's school, waiting for him to come out. From my vantage point, I could look inside the building. The sound of a bell indicated that school was out, and soon a stampede of children would stream through those gates of freedom, but it always seemed that Connor was one of the last ones.

When he finally came out, he was talking to one of his friends. He was distracted and not paying attention to anything around him. He just stood there talking away. I placed both my hands around my mouth to amplify and direct my voice better. Once he heard me calling his name, he instantly turned and started to run my direction with his hands in the air waving. He flew into my arms and as I kissed the top of his head I asked,

"Hey buddy, how was school?"

While he was talking about his day, we started to walk towards the Sixth-Grade center that was located on the opposite side of the parking lot. My eyes were fixated on two doors on the side of the building from where Dane would be coming out from. A stream of youngsters burst through the doors, screaming, jumping, running around, neglecting the calls from parents. As wild, uncontrollable young animals without purpose they continued to run everywhere. Onto the sidewalk, on the road, and over the grass field. Dane's white blond hair was recognizable from miles away, like the beacon of a lighthouse providing direction for ships at night. He knew I was going to be here and as soon as he came out, he started to scan the area in search of me. I called his name,

"Dane!"

He recognized the sound of my voice immediately. He turned his little head like a hawk that suddenly noticed his prey. His eyes locked, recognizing, smiling, and then running as fast as his little legs could run. With his arms spread wide open, he was accelerating over the concrete, his backpack bouncing on his back. It seemed he was planning to take off for flight. He ran into my arms, almost knocking me over. With a big smile on his face, he looked up at me with those large green eyes that no one could resist.

"Papa!" he yelled joyfully, squeezing me as hard as he could.

I cupped his face between my hands, kissed his bright blond hair.

"Hey sweetie. Did you have a good day at school?" I asked.

He locked both his arms around my neck and would not let go. I picked him up with ease, planted him on my right side, and as he laid his precious little head on my shoulder, I leaned my head towards him to lock it in place. I turned around, grabbed Connor's hand and we all walked to the truck. We were surrounded by herds of kids with parents that were walking in all kinds of directions. Dane remained silent and just enjoyed the comfort of clinging on to me.

On our way home, I told the boys that mama was not feeling well and that we all should be quiet when we got there. It was amazing to see how well the boys were doing with all that was going on in their little lives. From the moment I told them that their mama had cancer, they never questioned anything. I continued to have frequent conversations with them about what was going on and what we were doing. I knew they had all the information like everyone else. Sometimes they would have questions, and they would always ask me, not Becky. All they did around her was love her, be with her, and snuggle with her.

When we got home, they walked softly through the hallway to drop their bags off in their room. Before they got halfway through the hallway, a voice came from our bedroom.

"Who is there sneaking through the hallway?" Becky said.

"Are those my two sweetheart boys?"

They dropped their bags in the hallway like a sack of potatoes, increased their speed and climbed onto our bed, sandwiching Becky with arms around her and placing kisses all over her face. She radiated love and joy to her two boys, loving them unconditionally. Connor and Dane just laid there, nestling right next to her. Connor suddenly looked up and asked,

"Can we play a game on the Xbox?"

"I don't mind," I said.

"Okay," Becky said, "but only for one hour guys."

Since Becky was not feeling too well, I made some chicken noodle soup for dinner. Since we changed our diet to all organic, natural, and unprocessed foods, I spent much more time in the kitchen than ever before. Eating healthy was not only expensive, it was also very time consuming since you are using only fresh ingredients.

I placed the bowls with soup on the dining room table for the boys, accompanied by some grilled cheese sandwiches. The silence at the table confirmed that they were enjoying it. It always makes me feel good to see them eat the food I made. It meant they like it, and that is the biggest compliment I could ever get.

I placed Becky's bowl with a piece of toast on a bed-tray, so she could have dinner in bed. She was sitting upright reading her book, her reading glasses on the tip of her nose. She looked up from her story, glanced over the edges of her glasses, and smiled. She smoothly closed her book and placed it right next to her on the bed, then tapped both hands on her lap, telling me to place the tray right there.

"Thank you, sweetie," she said while grabbing the spoon and eating the warm goodness. "I am sure this will make me feel better soon," she added.

"I am going to check on the boys real quick, Sugar," I said, "I will be right back."

The boys were already done with their food and asked if they could have more.

"Of course," I said, as I started to fill their bowls with more soup.

I turned the corner from the hallway into our bedroom. Becky had stopped eating, although the tray was still in front of her, the soup bowl in the middle was still full, toast untouched, her face ashen, her lips pale.

"Not feeling so well babe," she stated without moving her body, her hand still holding on to the spoon.

"Really dizzy," she added.

I decided to get some vital signs on her. Her blood pressure was in the low 90s, and her heart rate was over 130s. I knew I had to take her into the emergency room, but before we took off, I sat down with the boys to explain what was going on. I did not want them to be confused about anything or to have any questions whatsoever.

I picked up Becky in my arms.

"No honey. Don't," she instructed me, but I knew she was too weak.

She was feeling miserable, and she was dizzy. I could carry her anywhere in the world if I needed to.

"I love you babe" was my only reaction to her statement.

As I secured her in my arms, she curled up closer to my body. She placed her head on my shoulder and let me be the knight I was supposed to be for her.

The night was bright, the stars started to pop up in the dark cover. The moon was big and causing this bluish glow on everything outside. The air still felt like glue on your skin. Interstate 35 was calm at this time of night. Becky sat next to me, staring at the road, holding my hand, not saying much. I knew she was not feeling well.

"I am going to call ahead sweetie," I said, "to see how busy they are."

A soft "Okay" came from her lips without moving anything else than absolutely needed to say those words.

"We have about twenty people in the waiting room," the charge nurse said.

"You might be better off to go to Mercy West. They only have two patients right now."

"Who is the doc over there?" I asked.

"It's Gerdis," she responded.

It was one of the docs that has been around for quite a long time. He must have been with our ER team for over ten years. I worked with him several times and respected him.

"Okay," I told the charge nurse, "I will head over there."

Since the west location was only about fifteen minutes farther, I determined it was worth the extra driving time.

"Honey," I told Becky, "I am taking you to the west location since downtown is packed right now, okay?"

"Mhmh," Becky just hummed to confirm.

The wheels of my truck made a delicate squeak as I turned onto the newly poured concrete of the parking lot, conveniently located right in front of the emergency department entrance. The west location was built not that long ago, so everything was still very new. There were only two more cars parked outside.

"Looks like they were right," I said softly while I parked my truck right under the light-pole that provided bright illumination. After the truck came to a complete stop, I turned off the engine, looked at Becky and said,

"Stay right here babe, I am going to get you a wheelchair."

The receptionist behind the desk recognized me. She apparently also worked frequently at the downtown hospital.

"They already called me from the main ER that you would be coming," she stated.

"Okay," I responded, "I am just getting a wheelchair for my wife and I will be back."

"Do you need any help?" she asked.

"No, I am good," I said as I pushed the wheelchair through the sliding doors.

I placed it along the truck, facing Becky's door, pushed the two metal levers down to apply the brakes. Carefully I opened the passenger door and helped Becky get into the wheelchair.

"Thank you, sweetie," she said as she sat down.

The check in process was fast and simple. Within ten minutes we were on our way to a room. While Becky was sitting on the edge of the bed, I helped her put on the hospital gown. After she laid down, I covered her with blankets, my eyes locked onto hers. Knowing she was always cold, I inquired,

"Are you warm enough honey?"

She confirmed with a nod and, "I am good for now. Thank you, babe."

After I snuggled the blankets around her, I sat down next to her, holding her hand.

A soft knock on the door and as it opened, a kind female voice introduced herself as the nurse. She was in her mid-twenties, short blond hair, tall and skinny. I recognized her; she was a new nurse. Not that long ago, she was still in training at the main ER. After she completed a set of vital signs, I told her that I had seen her in the main ER. She smiled and confirmed that she was recently released from training.

She explained the standard routine in the ER. An IV would be placed for fluids, and blood drawn for the lab. When she noticed that Becky had a port, she seemed uncomfortable accessing it. Establishing a port access for an IV and bloodwork can be intimidating for new nurses. It is more a matter of practice than anything else, but I remembered when I was a new nurse and had to access a port for the first time, I was really uncomfortable doing it.

"Are you not comfortable with accessing a port?" I asked her since I clearly noticed the fear in her eyes.

"Well," she said, "I have not done many of them yet," she honestly admitted.

"You can just do a normal IV in my arm," Becky said, since she also noticed the nurse was hesitant about it.

"I really don't care, and I have great veins. The port is still a little tender anyway."

The relief was clearly noticeable. "Are you sure?" the nurse asked.

Becky nodded and confirmed. "Sure, it's no problem at all."

"I will be right back," she told us as she left the room, "I need to get some supplies."

I looked at Becky and asked her if she was sure about not using the port.

"It's fine honey," she responded, "It does not make a difference to me if she uses my arm or the port."

The ER nurse returned with the supplies she needed. She pulled the metal table with small wheels closer and placed several items on top of it. She walked over to a cabinet, next to the bed, opened the drawer and while she got some IV supplies, she confirmed,

"Are you sure you are ok with me not using your port?"

"Whatever you are more comfortable with," Becky said, "my arm or the port."

The nurse smiled as she started to get ready.

He was sitting on the rolling stool, straight back, captivated by the sheets of papers he was holding in his hands, flipping from one page to the other, and then back again. He was wearing green surgical scrubs with a white coat. All ER-providers had access to the physician lounge in the hospital where they were not only provided with food and beverages, but also bright green surgical scrubs to wear. The white coat was his own. He was one of the few that still wore one.

I always assumed he was military because of his immaculate and particularly sequenced approach for patient assessments. Although he never denied nor confirmed, his overall appearance radiated military. He had an unexpected, amazing dry sense of humor. He could make remarks and everyone would burst out in tears of laughter, but he would not move a muscle or show any type of emotion.

I think that most of the ER nurses enjoyed working with him since he was very precise in his progression of patient assessment. Patient care was always on top of his list of priorities.

"If there is only one thing we can do for our patients, it is to control their pain," he told me once.

"Regardless of all other things, it is our duty to assure the patient is comfortable without any hardship from pain."

He had an impressive ability to analyze the true patients' condition and needs, regardless of their subjective complaints and concerns.

Silence had taken over the room while he continued to shuffle through the papers that were clearly the reports from Becky's lab work. You could hear a soft "mhmm" sound coming from him with a gentle nod. We were staring at him as if we were bewitched by his presence.

"Okay," he suddenly burst out, breaking the silence.

He detached his attention from his papers and looked at Becky. Both hands resting in his lap, holding on to the report. He took a deep breath in, his chest expanding,

"Becky, I am sorry that you have to be here tonight, and I am very sorry for your recently discovered condition."

The undertone of true care was undeniably present.

"But I know you are in the very capable and caring hands of your husband."

He reached in his pocket from the white coat and pulled out a stethoscope.

"Let me first look at you."

I knew the exact progression he would follow for his assessment of the patient. From lung sounds, to heart sounds and rhythm, followed by abdominal sounds. After he folded up his stethoscope and put it back in his coat pocket, he would use the otoscope to look into her ears, her throat and use it for a pupillary reaction.

As he satisfactorily completed his mission, he sat back onto the stool, with both his hands back onto his lap.

"All your lab results look normal," he started, "some of your electrolytes are off, indicating that you are possibly dehydrated causing the dizziness."

As he continued to explain the importance of fluid status in any human being, but especially when a person is sick, I noticed that Becky was very attentive to what he was saying. She was nodding frequently and focused on his words.

As usual he was almost painstakingly detailed, but he wanted to make sure that Becky understood. As a nurse, but especially as a husband, I really appreciated his detailed explanation and the time he was spending with her, ensuring that Becky understood the situation and the actions that could be taken to avoid this from occurring again. He clarified to her that she should be avoiding any type of caffeine since it actually caused dehydration.

"So coffee, tea, and dark sodas should not be on your list," he confirmed.

He also explained that whenever a person's system is battling a disease, it is important to eliminate any possibility for dehydration.

"Your system is trying to fight this cancer inside of you, and it will be imperative to eradicate any toxin possible to allow your body to focus on the war with cancer and healing damaged tissues." A very clear, constructive, and understandable clarification, I thought.

"So, we are going to get some fluids going and give you some anti-dizziness medicine and see how you do in a couple of hours, okay?" he concluded.

"That sounds good," Becky confirmed.

The nurse returned and, as she walked over to the IV-pump, she explained that,

"I am going to change the settings so the fluids run in a little faster."

She pushed on different buttons that gave short beeping sounds to confirm settings. The slow drip rate suddenly became faster, and the drip-container showed a consistent stream of fluids instead of dripping.

Throughout the evening, Becky continued to improve and she was released from the emergency department later that night. When we arrived at home, it was late, both boys had already been asleep for hours. They had school the next day, so we normally had them in bed around eight o'clock.

Lisa was asleep on the couch. I had asked her to come over and take care of Connor and Dane while Becky and I were going to the ER. She arrived right before we left the house.

Her hair was bewildered like a wild cave woman, her face wrinkled from resting her head on the armrest of the couch. Hugs and kisses were exchanged as she left our home.

Becky and I checked on the boys together, standing in the doorway, I was leaning against the doorpost, Becky leaning against me, my arm around her. We just stood there and watched them sleep, our boys. I turned my head towards Becky, observed the radiance from her eyes, pride, love, and fear. My chest felt heavy, my soul wept. Holding back my tears, I placed a delicate kiss on her temple followed by a soft

"I love you."

She turned her head, her glittering eyes stared at me. She placed her right hand on my cheek, stood on the tip of her toes to reach my lips, kissed, and released.

"Thank you for taking care of me," she said, "I love you."

We crawled in our bed, Becky on her right side, my left arm over her body, my right arm under her pillow, my face was in the corner of her head and neck, smelling her hair, her skin; a pleasant addicting intoxication.

Eight

The sun had just broken through the horizon. It was early morning and everyone was still asleep. The air outside still pleasant, almost like a fresh crisp spring morning that created small drops of dew on every blade of grass. The sticky humid air that hangs on to your skin and made breathing difficult, because of the thick sultry heaviness, was still far from here. I had a great night of continuous sleep, and it seemed that Becky experienced the same as she was still comfortably snoozing. It warmed my heart to see her sleep well.

Quietly, I left our bedroom, and as I gently closed our door, a soft squeak from the hinges caused my heart to skip a beat. Although the sound was noticeable, it did not disturb her sleep. I tip-toed through the hallway, into the sleeping quarters of the boys. Their floor was like a minefield of toys, Lego's, dinky toys, and other skin penetrating items. I had to wake them up as they needed to get ready for school.

After they attacked and devoured the homemade breakfast burritos like hungry dogs, they grabbed their backpacks and got ready for school. Becky was still sound asleep when we left, I placed a little sticky note on her nightstand:

'Taking the boys to school. Be back in 20 minutes. Love you. xoxoxo.'

After I had dropped off the boys at school, I tried to sneak back into the house. I opened the front door with a superior delicacy, to ensure silence would be maintained. As I stepped into the house, I glanced up the seven steps that lead to the living room area, and there she was, standing at the top with a big smile,

"Morning sweetie," she welcomed me back home.

I walked up the stairs and as I arrived next to her, I placed a soft kiss on her lips.

"Let me make you some breakfast, babe" I said.

The sun started to make its journey along the bright blue sky, but it was still too early for it to mold the air into a humid stickiness. Since it was such a pleasant morning, we opened most of the windows to get some fresh air flowing through the house. Becky was sitting outside enjoying a nice cup of warm green tea. She had just finished some scrambled eggs and grits. Personally, I detested the taste and texture of grits, but it was one of her favorites. We were blessed with a grocery store that had a large organic section, so Becky was pleased that they had organic grits.

I was doing some dishes by hand since the dishwasher was full and still running. As I stood there, I watched Becky through the kitchen window. She was sitting on our wicker loveseat, sipping her green tea. At that moment I was unaware of events that would unfold soon. If I had known what was brewing amongst some family members, I would have tried to alter the path they were on.

Later that morning, Becky and I were confronted with an episode where pain, stress, fear, and misunderstanding had caused some family members to act in an unexplainable and unexpectedly harsh manner. It was understandable that the diagnosis of lung cancer was a shock to everyone. Everyone was under a lot of stress. Every person also has a different coping mechanism to deal with devastating news. Some people might flee the situation by avoiding exposure to the environment, some might sit quietly in a chair while others cry out loud. Others might want to blame someone or something for their misery.

No matter the reasoning, when this occurs in a family setting, it might cause a massive rupture in the family structure that will be difficult, if at all, to repair. No matter what, the scars of such actions will never completely disappear. The destruction of the tenants of trust will be most likely irreparable.

That morning, Becky and I faced such a catastrophic situation where misunderstanding, stress, and miscommunication caused an unneeded disaster. Some family members questioned my character and attempted to discredit me as a person, but they underestimated the strong and solid relationship Becky and I had .

While I was being attacked, Becky determined that there was no other solution than to ask them to leave our house. It caused an unnecessary awkward situation for everyone.

When Becky and I were confronted with this behavior, it felt like a slap in the face. We were shocked and confused. Both of us never expected this to happen. These were unjustified attacks and caused unneeded confusion, pain, and sadness for all of us.

Later that night, after all the commotion settled, Becky and I were sitting on our seat outside on the deck. The sun was dark red, falling through a purple blanket, sinking into the unknown depths of the horizon. Both boys were already in bed. The TV was on, volume soft, just some background noise. Today was a crazy day full of unexpected madness. We both were quite confused about the actions that took place that morning. As we were exchanging thoughts, Becky's left eye was blinking more than the other.

"Do you have something in your eye sweetie?" I asked.

She denied anything in her eye, but she told me that she was seeing a blind spot in the center of her vision field. After I looked into her eye and did not find anything, we brushed it off as maybe stress from today.

"If it is still here tomorrow, we will call Doctor Freeman," Becky said.

The night settled over the hot warm day with a clear dark cloak. The moon seemed amazingly large, bright and perfectly round. The dark calmness provided an eerie sense of peace after this day that was filled with unwanted and unexpected turmoil. Becky fell asleep within minutes after we laid our bodies to rest. The emotional stress from the day caused an increased drainage on her already low energy supply.

She was comfortably on her favorite side, her breathing deep and calm, evenly paced. My eyes fixated on the ceiling, resting on my back, my hands interlocked and placed on my stomach. My mind explored the events of the day, replaying them over and over on the screen of my consciousness. While the images appeared before me, I understood that we all were having a difficult time with the newly discovered disease Becky was facing. Cancer was not on anyone's horizon.

It is human nature to try to find a 'why' and to blame someone for their misery. That was the only reason I could come up with for their actions. They were mad, upset, confused, and had to blame someone for their discomfort. We have a saying in the Netherlands that 'when a cat gets pushed into a narrow corner, it will make weird jumps to get out of it'. This seemed applicable in this situation, and this 'cat' for sure made some really weird jumps. Nevertheless, my heart felt heavy, filled with sadness, wishing this had never happened.

I had just gotten off the phone with Doctor Freeman, Becky's eye was not doing any better, actually, she explained, it was a little worse. It seemed that the black spot was getting bigger compared to yesterday. This was a concerning development, so I decided that it was time to inform Doctor Freeman of this situation.

"It is imperative to get her eye evaluated as soon as possible by a specialist," he instructed me.

He promised that he would call the Wolfe Eye clinic in West Des Moines to get an appointment with one of the ophthalmologists for further evaluation and possible treatment of this problem.

Becky was sitting outside, enjoying the weather. It was a pleasant day, not too hot or humid. She was sitting outside, working on her rug. I made her some fruit juice with apple, pear, beets, and carrots, that was her favorite. I placed the glass, filled with nature's healing nectar, on the table in front of her.

"Here you go sweetie," I said.

Becky looked up from her rug without moving her head, just her eyes staring at me right over the edge of her reading glasses that were positioned on the tip of her nose. A big smile welcomed the arrival of the freshly pressed drink.

"Thank you, babe," she said.

Becky enjoyed rug-hooking and spent many hours making the most elaborate rugs. Many of them were designed from pictures of the boys. Her mother had been rug-hooking for as long as I can remember, and she had gotten all her daughters addicted to this activity.

Before I could sit down and explain my conversation with Doctor Freeman, my phone rang. It was the Wolfe Eye clinic. They had an opening later this afternoon and wanted to know if Becky could come in for some testing to determine the cause of the blind spot in her eye. I placed my hand on the bottom of my phone and whispered to Becky,

"They want to see you this afternoon for your eye. You ok with that?"

Becky confirmed, with a big nod and a soft, but excited, "Yes."

Upon our arrival at the eye clinic, we sat down to fill out the required paperwork. After I completed the forms for Becky, I walked over to the front desk, and gave them to the young lady behind the counter. She informed me that,

"Someone will call her back soon."

I smiled and nodded.

We were sitting at the far end of the waiting room where Becky was talking to an older couple. She introduced me to them and explained that he had been dealing with cancer also, and that he had been getting high vitamin C infusions in Mexico. I sat down next to Becky, and as always, she grabbed my hand to hold on to.

They were an older couple, in their mid-sixties. He had those bushy grey eyebrows that jumped with every movement of his face. No facial hair, but still some hair on top, white gray but appropriate for his age. She had long dark blond hair with many gray strands. It seemed that she had tried to cover up her white silver hair before, since a clear demarcation of hair coloring was noticeable about 3 inches from the scalp.

They still seemed very much in love; you could hear it in their tone of voice when they talked to each other, it was saturated with tenderness. They touched each other frequently, gentle subtle taps on arms or legs filled with passion. Most of all, when they looked at each other, their eyes revealed their higher connection. They had a history but never left the other behind.

He told us that he had been struggling with cancer for many years, but that he started to go to Mexico for high vitamin C infusions. He went to Mexico, he explained, because getting vitamin C infusions in America was almost impossible. He was adamant about the positive impact these infusions had on his overall health. He was cancer-free now for many years and he was convinced that they helped him defeat cancer.

I explained to him about all my personal research about diets, glyconutrients, and juicing. He wanted to make sure we would not leave anything untouched.

"You will be amazed," he said, "when you discover what other countries incorporate in the treatment of cancer. They embrace holistic treatments as part of the overall attack to beat cancer."

He was probably unaware of the spark he lit up inside of me to continue my research, now even more aggressively than before. When we were called back by the nurse, we shook hands, his grip was firm but comfortable. I placed my left hand on the back of his hand that was already in the shaking, to assure he knew how much I appreciated his time, his openness and honesty.

The technician told Becky to place her chin on top of the plastic support device of the large machine. He explained that the optical camera would scan her retina. Becky leaned slightly forward, placed her chin in the white plastic cup-looking device and leaned her forehead onto support bar.

"Look straight ahead into the light," he said as a bright light came from the machine, aiming into Becky's eye.

Becky was silent, staring aimlessly into the machine, not moving.

"After the scan," he explained as he was making adjustments to the machine, "I will also take some pictures of your eye, so continue to look forward and you will see several bright flashes."

The engine inside this large apparatus made a buzzing sound. As the noise intensified, the technician warned that there would be several bright flashes. Almost immediately the first flash lit up most of the room. After several more, he told us,

"Ok, we are done here."

We left the room and he guided us through a labyrinth of hallways to another room. He opened the door and stood in the opening and waved his hand inward.

"Just have a seat here and the doctor will be with you in a moment, after he analyzes the images."

This room had a large chair in the middle that looked almost like a dentist chair. Becky decided to sit with me on the chairs that were placed to the side.

After the nurse completed the input of some additional health information into the computer system, she explained that she would inform the ophthalmologist that we were ready.

After introductions, he sat down and pulled up the images on his computer screen. In detail he explained what we were looking at. There were black and white layers on the screen. These were the layers of Becky's retina of her left eye. He used his pen to tap on the screen, and both Becky and I were staring, almost hypnotized, at these images. The layers seemed all the same and pretty much straight on top of each other. There was one area, where there was a large bump in the middle of these layers. This bump, according to the ophthalmologist, was the metastasis of the cancer to the retina of the eye. It had nestled itself within the layers causing the blind spot in Becky's vision.

Just like that, out of the blue, a slap in your face. The cancer was now showing up in her eye. We knew that the cancer had spread throughout her body, but as far as we knew, it was in the lung and on the bones. The appearance of cancer in her eye was a rude awakening. It had traveled to her eye, so now it was very close to her brain. We both wondered if it anywhere else in her head we could not see yet?

Becky did not move, she just kept staring at the screen as if the news of cancer flew right past her and that the news did not have any impact on her. But her hand, that was holding mine, became stronger in her grip. I knew she was worried and scared. The fear that this was just the beginning of an uncontrollable infestation of cancer that would take over her whole body soon. The fear that this cancer could be popping up in different locations; an unruly and violent spread of the disease leaving no healthy tissue behind to result in a rapidly ending road.

The ophthalmologist explained that he had treated this before in other patients, and that he had a good response by injecting a medication called Avastin into the eyeball itself.

"This medication prevents the growth of blood vessels to the cancer," he explained, "thus killing it by means of starvation."

He would perform this procedure on a monthly basis until the tumor had diminished. Sometimes radiation would also be needed to control it.

"So, you are going to stick a needle in my eye?" Becky asked.

The vibration in her voice explained the fear she had for such a procedure.

He explained that he would first numb her eye with some eye-drops, and that she would not feel anything. All she had to do was to make sure to keep her eye still. With marked hesitation in her voice, she confirmed to the treatment. While the nurse collected all the needed equipment and medication, he told Becky to sit still in the chair and stare at a spot on the wall to the right.

"Hang on," she said, reaching out her hand towards me, making a gripping movement with her fingers.

"Come here sweetie," she told me.

I moved my chair right next to the one Becky was sitting in, grabbing and holding her hand. My eyes were only fixed on her, our hands engaged, our fingers intertwined. She laid her head down on the headrest of the chair. After the nurse placed several drops in her eye, the eye became numb. The ophthalmologist moved closer, holding the syringe with the medicine in his right hand, talking to Becky all the time, explaining what he was going to do, trying to comfort her.

She continued to hold my hand with an increased grip, her knuckles white. Her body tensed, her eyes locked onto a small frame on the wall, not speaking, shallow breathing, increased rhythm, but shallow. As he instructed her to keep looking at that frame and to not blink, his right hand moved closer to her eye. Her grip became stronger in my hand. He placed the needle closer and with a gentle but swift move, the metal stick sank into her eyeball. She did not blink, did not deviate from her fixation point, and did not move a muscle. As the needle was inserted into her eye, he gradually pushed the plunger with his thumb, allowing the medicine to penetrate inside of her eye.

Within seconds, he meticulously removed the syringe with the needle, and as it departed Becky's eye, he said,

"All done."

"Really? Already? Can I move?" Becky asked, almost shocked about how fast this went. He assured her she was done, and as she looked at him with some disbelief, but before she could say anything he explained,

"You did great. You did not move at all."

Her face lit up, like a child receiving an unexpected present, big smile, eyes sparkling. Relieved it was over and done with, she sighed, "Good."

We were back home from the eye clinic before dinner time. While Lisa and Becky were talking out back on the deck, I started to make dinner. Something simple was on the menu for tonight: tomato soup with grilled cheese sandwiches. As usual I made a fresh fruit juice for Becky, but since the boys liked it too, I always made plenty for everyone. The boys were playing a game on the Xbox and I could hear their voices coming from the living room. I always made grilled cheese sandwiches in a frying pan, and the moment I placed the first couple of sandwiches in the hot butter, Dane yelled excited from the living room.

"Are you making grilled cheese, Papa?"

He loved the way I made grilled cheese sandwiches.

"Yes sweetie," I said, "I will let you know when it is ready."

As I started to put placemats and silverware on the table, both Becky and Lisa came inside. Lisa was going home, so she gave everyone a hug and kiss. Becky sat down with the boys in the living room until I was done putting the soup and sandwiches on the table.

One of the Dutch favorites, is to eat a grilled cheese sandwich with curry-ketchup. In the Netherlands, you can just buy a bottle of this at the grocery store, but since it was unknown here in America, I made it myself. It is quite simple, just mix some curry seasoning with ketchup.

I started to pour the soup into bowls and placed them on the dining room table. A large stack of grilled cheese sandwiches was placed on top of each other on a large plate in the middle, accompanied by a large bowl of homemade 'curry-ketchup'.

I called for all to come for dinner. We would always try to have a sit-down dinner with everyone in the evening. It provided for time together as a family to talk about the day and things that were going on. No TV, no phones, just food and conversation. Tonight, was one of those nights that Becky felt pretty good to be with us at the dining room table. Although she did not eat much, we were all happy to have her join us.

During dinner, Dane explained that he had signed up at school to be the class president and that he would have a presentation the next day. He was very excited about it and wanted us both to come.

Nine

The sidewalks were infested with parents walking with their children. Some kids were holding their parents' hands, while others were uncontrollably running all over sidewalks, the grass, and the parking lot. They were all streaming towards the front doors of the school building. Like cattle being corralled into their pens. The flow through the portals caused humans, big and small, to slow down, to line up outside and gradually enter the structure.

Once inside, everyone was directed to the school gym, where bleachers were set up for the parents and benches on the floor for the kids. Every child that wanted to be a delegate for their class was doing a promotional speech that morning to entice those who would be voting the following week to elect their class representatives.

I was walking with Dane through the crowds to get to the school gym. Becky was upset she couldn't come with us, but she was just not feeling well enough to come along. As we entered the school gym, Dane was directed to the center to sit with the other children. I wrapped him in my arms, gave him a kiss and whispered in his ear,

"You will do great."

He smiled, squeezed his arms tight around my neck, and said,

"I love you Papa."

He warmed my heart, I kissed him again,

"Love you too buddy," and off he went to sit with the others.

As I made my way through the crowds to find a good spot on one of the bleachers, many stopped me and asked how 'things' were. A really awkward question. I know that people asked it to show their concern and their compassion for the situation, but 'things' were horrible. Besides, this would not be the right moment to go into a discussion about the disease that was possibly slowly killing my sweetheart. I did appreciate the thought, but after many of the same questions, about 'things' I wanted to fade away in the masses, to become invisible.

I noticed a good spot on the top of the bleachers. From there I had a great view of the stage where they would be giving their promotional speeches. I planted myself victoriously on my found location and waited for the event to start.

It was Dane's turn after several other kids spoke. As he walked towards the stage, I felt an enormous sense of pride. Here was my little guy, only ten years old, going on stage to give a speech to a full school gym about why his classmates should vote for him to become the next class president. Something I would not have done when I was his age.

He was determined about his mission, a quality you did not see often in humans. I could feel the excitement growing inside me. As he stepped on stage, many people clapped, but I am sure I was the loudest. He had his speech written down, and with it in his hand, he walked towards the microphone.

All alone he stood there on that big platform. The teacher adjusted the microphone to his height. Dane looked up. I noticed that his eyes were searching for me. I raised my hand, and when he saw me, he smiled. His left hand waved at me from the hip. Without hesitation he started to speak, his voice loud and clear.

"My name is Dane Slootheer…"

He continued to explain the things he would do if he were elected class president.

As his speech continued, he shifted gears and informed all who were there about the main reason for him to become class president.

"My mom just got back from the hospital," he said, "and she has just been diagnosed with cancer. I know she will get better, but I want to do the best I can do and make her proud."

The words flowing from his lips caused an emotional shake inside my heart. My hand went to my mouth, and as I placed it over my lips, I softly whispered,

"Oh sweetie..."

I could feel tears welling up inside me and before I could do anything, they escaped. I closed my eyes, trying to push back my tears, but this flow of emotion was fierce and stronger than my will.

After his speech was done, everyone was applauding. I stood up, again clapping louder than anyone there, wiping my tears. For most people there, this was just a moment in time, but to me it was locked into my heart for a lifetime. The school principal was standing at the bottom of the bleachers, staring at me. He knew what was going on, and he knew that this would hit me right in the heart. He smiled and nodded, acknowledging his understanding.

The kids were released after all the speeches were done. Dane came running over as I started to make my way down from the bleachers. I welcomed him with both my arms spread wide open, and as I crouched down, he flew into my arms. My lips placed a kiss on his cheek, I looked him in the eyes, and said,

"I am so proud of you buddy, that was an awesome speech."

He smiled and hugged me. "You liked it?" he asked.

"It was the best speech I ever heard," I exclaimed while still pushing back the tears.

We both walked out of the school gym, towards his class. Before releasing him into the classroom, I squatted down, surrounded him with my arms and squeezed him tightly. He wrapped his arms around my neck and placed his soft cheek against mine.

"I love you buddy, see you after school," I told him.

"Love you too Papa," he answered as he ran into the classroom, looking at me and waved his little hand in the air.

While I walked through the hallways, dodging kids left and right, I realized that it would have been great for Dane if Becky would have been able to be there and to hear his speech. He worked hard on it, and I know he really wanted his Mama there, but I wondered how Becky would have handled it. Maybe it would have been too much for her, too emotional. This was an anxious time for all of us. We were all emotionally hyped and uncertain about the future.

Becky was sitting straight up in bed, on the phone talking to someone. Her voice sounded excited, and as I walked in the bedroom, she waved her hand at me to come over. While she finished up the conversation, she grabbed my hand. I sat down next to her on the bed, facing her.

"Ok, thank you so much, we will see you then."

She hung up the phone and looked at me with a big smile.

"Well, honey," she said, "that was Doctor Freeman. He told me that the results are back from the biopsy, and although we normally do not like mutations, this time it is a good thing."

That was really great news. The results from the biopsy showed that there was an EGFR gene mutation, causing the cancer cells to grow rapidly. EGFR stands for Epidermal Growth Factor Receptor, and when there is a mutation it will cause the epidermal cells, or skin cells, to grow faster than normal; the very basis for cancer to exist, the uncontrollable growth of cells. The good news was that this type of mutation is controllable with oral 'gene-targeted' medication. This oral medication would influence the EGFR gene and stop, or at least slow down, the gene that was causing the abnormal growth of cells. This medication would still have plenty of side-effects, but much less when compared to conventional chemotherapy. The ultimate goal would be to stop the cancer cells from growing.

There was another important benefit of using this oral medication first. As Doctor Freeman explained during our initial meeting with him, that cancer will eventually find a way around the medication and it will proceed to proliferate and grow bigger.

"Cancer is very unpredictable," Freeman explained, "and you might think you are doing well, just to come to the realization that it is suddenly growing again, or it starts to appear in other locations."

If cancer found a way around this gene-targeting medication, there would be two more treatments options; two different types of chemotherapy. So that was great news that we had been hoping for.

Since this was a unique medication and had to come from a specialty pharmacy, Doctor Freeman was going to order it. The cost was astronomical, $7,000 per month, but with the insurance we had, our copay was $150 per month. Doctor Freeman also wanted to have a follow-up appointment thirty days after Becky started with this new treatment to see how intense the side-effects were.

Since Becky had a lot of metastases to the bone, there was an increased risk that her bones could become brittle and there was an increased risk for fractures. Doctor Freeman wanted to start with a bone-strengthening medication.

The initial scans and MRIs showed cancer in the lung, lymphatic system, hipbone and along the vertebrae of the spine. No other metastases were found. Although it is common for lung cancer to spread to the liver and brain, Becky was not showing any activity in either.

It is amazing to realize how we take life for granted. Most of us assume we will live to grow old and see our children become adults and have their own families. Not many realize that it can be snatched away in a heartbeat. Only the few lucky ones will be able to view the world through old worn windows. It is sad to discover that something disastrous has to happen before we are shaken enough to appreciate what we have today.

Becky and I were no different than most. We never expected any of this to happen. We had plans: travel plans, business plans, young children that were growing up. A catastrophic disease such as cancer was far from our reality, yet it arrived with a vengeance. The road we were on was sunny and without too many obstacles. Of course, our relationship had some bumps here and there, but we figured it out. No matter how mad or upset anyone was, we would never leave the house or go to bed without saying 'I love you'.

This first month after the diagnosis of stage IV cancer was like a wild roller coaster ride. We were strapped into our seats on this mandatory gruesome journey. Becky and I grew closer. We knew each other, we were connected as not many would understand. Our tight bond was welded strong and any attack on that bond increased the foundation of our union.

We learned that we understood each other better without the spoken word, and although this disease was devastating, we grew stronger. I walked beside her in this dark night, holding her hand and trying to protect her from this monstrous storm that was so intense, it was ripping the flesh off our bones.

***

The smell of fried eggs, toasted bread, and freshly made coffee must have awakened Becky's senses. The boys were already at school, and when I returned from dropping them off, Becky was still comfortably sleeping. I snuck through the hallway towards our bedroom to peek around the doorpost. When observing her like this, in a comfortable sleep, I sensed peace and innocence, as if nothing had happened. It was as if she were just asleep, not on a battlefield fighting an unbalanced and unfair duel against an enemy that does not play according to the rules. My heart would always grow bigger when she was resting peacefully, she seemed so serene and pure. These moments were so precious, so innocent, so healing.

Sometimes when she was asleep, I would move close to her, silently, making sure her sleep would not be disturbed. I would raise my hands and aim my palms towards her. Concentrating on everything that was pure and good, I tried to let the heavenly goodness with healing forces flow through me and surround her with this divine blanket.

As I would feel the energy flowing through me, I focused on helping her cells heal with this immersion of positive waves. Tears would travel down my face, a flow of pure and clean emotion. My soul would wrap around her body, trying to suck out the blackness from this invader causing this slow, horrible death. These moments between us were never seen. No one needed to know. Although Becky was asleep, I knew, deep down she was aware. This was us together in its finest form.

Today was her birthday and breakfast would be delivered in bed. Some whole wheat toast and scrambled eggs the way she liked them, fluffy and moist. A glass of fresh pressed juice from apples, pears, carrots, and beets would accompany this birthday early morning meal. As I started to plate everything, she called me from our bedroom.

"Honey?"

"I am on my way sweetie," I responded.

I made sure everything was on the tray and walked to our bedroom. A warm smile welcomed my appearance. I flipped open the stands of the tray and placed it over her legs as she raised the head of the bed up. We had a Tempur-Pedic mattress with a powered base, so it was easy to raise and lower the head and foot end of the bed with the simple touch of a button.

Some breadcrumbs and about half of the scrambled eggs were left on the plate. Becky placed her fork down, tapped on her stomach and politely confirmed,

"That was great honey, but I am full."

Later that afternoon we went outside to sit on our deck and soak up some energizing warmth. Since Becky was forced to stay out of direct sunlight, a side effect from the new medicine, prolonged direct sunlight was not recommended. We were sitting in the shade of the large oak trees that were directly behind our house. Connor and Dane were running around in our backyard, making some kind of fort to keep the zombies out. The joy in Becky's eyes as she watched our boys playing in our backyard was a simple pleasure to observe.

Throughout the afternoon people stopped by to see Becky and wish her happy birthday. I knew how she must have felt. Even though she was smiling and talking with everyone as if nothing were wrong, she probably had the same question I had when we were celebrating my birthday just a few short months ago. Birthdays were just no longer the same when you, or someone you love, is staring the grim reaper in the eyes.

Connor's birthday was a month ago. I took him and his friends to play laser tag. Becky did not have the energy to be there, and although Connor had a blast with his friends, I knew it was not the same for him either. Today was just another day we tried to have fun and enjoy friends and family, but the darkness and somberness were always there breathing down our necks, assuring we would not forget that Becky was in a bloodshed clash with death itself.

A week after her birthday, we went to see Doctor Freeman for our monthly visit. After the check-in at the front desk, they would always draw some blood for analysis. While we were still sitting at the draw station, Doctor Freeman's nurse Angie came in. She was always very friendly, big smile, and a warm welcome. She was the right person for this job. She truly cared, and I am sure that working with oncology patients is not easy since you are always helping those that are facing death.

She was a single mom and her boys were about the same age as Connor and Dane. We would always discuss the things we did or planned on doing with the kids. While we were walking down the hallway to the exam room where we would meet Doctor Freeman, Angie walked in front of us, but often she would turn around, slow down and talk about anything while she was walking backwards. She was gifted in making people feel welcome and at home in an environment nobody wanted to be.

It seemed we always ended up in the same exam room, right next to Doctor Freeman's office. Angie left after she completed her assessment, and Doctor Freeman walked in within minutes. The big smile on his face made his eye squint just a bit, his hand reached out to shake ours,

"Good to see you both," he said.

He was excited since the discovery of the EGFR gene mutation, and he was very curious how Becky was responding in taking the oral gene-targeting medication; Tarceva. Sometimes people can have disastrous reactions, like severe diarrhea, constipation, severe acne, and many other skin problems. Becky had some abdominal discomfort with minor diarrhea, and dry skin patches, but besides that, the reaction to the medication was not that uncomfortable. He was pleased with these developments and explained that we would do a Zometa infusion today. This was the bone-strengthening IV medication.

"We will also order a new CT-scan for next month to see how things are," he told us.

The plan was to come back every month for a follow up with him, and a CT-scan every three months to restage the cancer and determine if it was responding well to the treatment. He seemed quite thrilled about how things had been faring over the last couple of months.

We were directed to go upstairs to the infusion center that was conveniently located right above Doctor Freeman's office. There were six private rooms with beds, and about twenty recliners for all those who needed an infusion of some sort. There were not many patients there when we arrived.

We walked through the hallway and followed the infusion nurse. She explained that we could have a private room if we wanted. Since it was our first time there, Becky preferred some privacy and confirmed that she would like to have a private room.

These rooms were a good sized one bedroom, with a single bed, a chair and table. Becky sat down on the edge of the bed and the nurse came back with the supplies to access her port and start the infusion of the bone-strengthening medication.

The nurse exposed the top right part of Becky's chest to visualize the placement of the port. It was triangle shaped and undeniably present just below Becky's collarbone. The pink color of the scar revealed the short history of the port placement procedure. Through the thin skin layer there were small bumps noticeable, these were strategically placed on the port for proper identification of where the penetration with the needle should occur.

After the nurse cleansed the skin, she removed a large bore needle, that was shaped in a ninety-degree angle, from the package. She held it between the thumb and index finger of her right hand while her left fingers were tapping and moving, almost like dancing, over the skin that was covering the device trying to find the correct location to push the needle into the port.

After she found the perfect position, she placed her index finger on top of it and started to bring the needle closer to Becky's skin. As she was ready to press it through, her index finger that was covering the spot, slowly moved from that area. The sharp metal tip was now almost touching Becky's skin. She warned Becky,

"Here we go ... big sharp poke ..."

A determined fast and controlled thrust pushed the needle through the skin and into the port. Becky had her face turned the opposite direction, with one eye closed, squeezing it so tight it was making wrinkles on that side of her face. She always had been terrified of needles. She was preparing herself for the worse, but her response of

"Oh, that's it?", clarified it was less painful that she expected.

Within 30 minutes, the small infusion bag was empty. It looked like a shriveled up, emptied out, old raisin, hanging there on a metal pole, hopelessly without any purpose left. The beeping sound from the IV-pump filled the room with an annoying tone that was increasing in intensity. Within minutes there was a soft but audible knock on the door. The nurse entered the room and turned off the IV pump. She detached the tubing from the port needle, as the attachment was removed, Becky was freed from her temporary imprisonment.

Becky's facial color was ashen. She looked gray and miserable. The nurse knew that Becky was not feeling well.

"Sometimes people have adverse reactions with this infusion, but it is quite normal," the nurse justified.

She was trying to calm Becky's apparent anxious and uncomfortable attitude. The nurse determined that some fluids and medicine would help make Becky feel better. She attached a new bag of saline fluids back to the port-needle that was still in place. While the clear fluid was running through the tubing at a rapid rate, an antiemetic medication was added to calm the nausea. Within fifteen minutes Becky confirmed that her nausea was dissipating, but regardless, the nurse decided that it would be best to infuse the whole bag of fluids.

"Some extra fluids always make you feel better," she told Becky while placing her hand softly on her shoulder.

The air outside provided for a comfortable warmth, with the sun, every now and then, breaking through the thin cloud layer. White, dispersed, stretched-out puffs of cotton were floating along the clear blue skies. The weather was becoming friendlier by the day, the intense heat had been replaced with a cooler atmosphere until we reached autumn, when the clouds would increase and release the usual thunderstorms with massive downpours. We were both sitting on the loveseat outside on our deck, holding hands silently, just enjoying the weather and each other. Out of the blue, Becky announced,

"I love you honey." Her hand gripped a little tighter around mine.

I opened my eyelids gradually and slowly turned my head towards her. Her eyes were still closed, soaking up the energizing warmth from the sun rays. She was smiling, almost smirking. She knew I was looking at her. I tilted my body towards hers, sealed our love with a gentle kiss, and confirmed my commitment to her as I confessed,

"I love you too babe."

These rare silent moments of peace provided an inexpressible sense of calmness and warmth. Both boys were still at school and I would have to break away from this wonderful experience soon. My eyes still aimed at my bride, I warned her about my upcoming departure.

"Ok honey," she responded,

"I am going to lay down and rest for a while anyway. I am still feeling a little off."

Ten

The house was wrapped in a blanket of complete silence when the boys and I walked through the front door. Even our little white fluffball dog, Mondavi, was nowhere to be found. The boys and I slithered through the house like navy seals, on our bare feet, gliding over the hardwood floor. As the leader of the squad team, I placed the back of my left hand on the right side of my mouth, turned my head over my left shoulder and whispered,

"Go and sit down in the living room, I am going to check on Mama."

Our bedroom door was halfway open, no sounds, only complete silence. Without disturbing the door, I peeked around the corner to discover Becky sound asleep in our bed. Mondavi was lying right next to her, his body along her upper legs, her hand placed over his small torso. I slowly backed up, and as my fingers wrapped around the bronze colored doorknob, I pulled it closed. I wanted to barricade any noise that might flow through the hallway to disturb her sleep. She needed her rest. I informed the troops on the couch that they had to be quiet since Mama was sleeping, but they could play on the Xbox if they wanted. *If they wanted?* What was I thinking? Of course, they wanted to play.

Chicken fried rice with peanut butter sauce, also known as sate-sauce in the Netherlands, was on the menu for tonight. It was fairly easy to make, good tasting, nutritious, and both the boys and Becky loved it. Over the last several months, I rejuvenated my cooking skills to ensure proper nutritional intake for all the hungry mouths in the house. Besides that, Becky and I determined that a healthy, non-GMO, all organic diet was going to be a part of the cancer treatment. We changed many aspects in regards to food preparation, grocery shopping, and food selection.

I opened the fridge to collect some organic vegetables, organic butter, and farm-raised, free-ranged chicken breast. Two large onions were already laying ready, waiting on the wood chopping-board, to be diced into small pieces. A voice from the bedroom arose,

"Honey?"

Becky's voice revealed a slight tremble with a distressed tone, it did not sound right. Immediately I stopped with whatever I was doing and moved at an increased speed toward the bedroom. Becky was sitting upright on the side of our bed. Her left arm straight along her body, holding herself upright, her fingers clenched around the edge of the mattress. Her right hand in a fist, knuckles tapping on her sternum in the center of her chest.

"I got a lot of pain, babe" she said, "right here."

She continued to rap her fist on her chest.

"It really hurts bad. Something is stabbing me right here."

She had some similar episodes of these unexplainable chest pains, but they were never this intense.

I remember that I used to have esophageal spasms myself and those were very painful. This pain Becky was having almost seemed the same. Back then, my physician told me to drink ice-cold water to relax and calm down the spasm. I wondered if that would work for her too.

"I am getting you a glass of cold water to drink, hang on babe," I said.

Within minutes I returned with a glass of water filled with little ice cubes, softly making clinking sounds as they hit against the sides of the glass. Becky was still sitting in the same position, she had not moved at all, her fist still knocking on the center of her chest. As soon as I walked in, she stopped the rhythmic banging and reached out for the glass of water. Her face showed a painful grimace, her eyes squinted.

As she started to lift the glass towards her mouth, small condensation drops rolled down along the sides of the glass, and as they became larger, gravity caused them to fall down into her lap. Her lips folded around the edge of the glass and she slowly started to pour the water down her throat. She took several big swigs, making loud gulping sounds. Half the water disappeared `into her body before she stopped, moved the glass away from her face, took several deep breaths and declared,

"I think it is getting better."

Her rapid breathing slowed down to a more controlled pattern. Her body no longer tensed up, and her shoulders started to relax. She raised her head and aimed her eyes at me,

"What is causing that pain? It really hurts bad."

She explained that it was a very sharp stabbing pain, that it was taking away her breath and made her whole body cramp up. Seemingly exhausted, drained from battling the pain, she laid back down in the bed.

"I am tired," she said, "I am going to rest for a little, ok babe?"

Still concerned about her, I asked "You ok honey?"

She nodded, and an obvious fake smile told me she was just that, 'just ok'. My lips connected to her forehead, and as I placed the palm of my hand on her cheek,

"I am going to feed the boys and I will be right back ok?"

"Okay honey" she said, as she turned on her side, pulled up her knees, and closed her eyes.

The boys were both sitting at the dining room table. A gentle steam arose from the plates filled with freshly made chicken fried rice. The fine smell of grilled vegetables, garlic, and chicken filled the house. Connor and Dane were sitting at the dining room table, across from each other, silently eating.

"Mama is not feeling so well guys, so I am going to check on her, okay?" I said and kissed them both on the tops of their heads.

"What's going on?" Connor asked as he broke the comfortable silence.

"Well," I started to explain, "Mama got some new medicine today, and it seems it is making her sick, and that is why she is not feeling well."

Both boys started to slow down their food intake as I was talking, focusing all their attention to what I was telling them.

I stepped into the hallway that leads to our bedroom and as I walked by the bathroom, I noticed the door was almost closed. I also saw that the light was on. Normally this door was wide open and the lights off. I tapped softly on the door.

"Honey?".

"Yes sweetie, just come in," Becky responded. She was sitting on the toilet seat.

"I just had to go pee, but now my chest pain is back again."

She was using her right fist tapping on her chest again, as if she was trying to knock it out of her.

"It is getting really bad honey."

She started to stand up, one hand placed on the counter, the other on the edge of the windowsill. Her facial color pale, breathing rapidly, her lips pursed.

"It hurts babe. It hurts really bad."

She was suffering, in serious distress, and as I walked towards her, she started to stumble forward in my direction. Her left hand was still on the counter, but her right hand was now flying through the air trying to reach me. I took one step to close the gap between us, and as I placed both my arms around her chest, her voice started to fade. "OH BABE, oh babe, the pain..."

Her facial tone disappeared, her knees gave in and buckled, her body went limp. I knew she was going to fall, so I entrapped her body within both my arms, securely around her chest, her motionless body in my arms. Sounds disappeared, the room faded, my vision focused on her, my movements slow but deliberate, as if I were in a slow-motion movie.

Her voice gone, her breathing stopped, her lifeless body in my arms, pressed against mine. Her head tumbled backwards with her eyes wide open staring at the ceiling. Her arms limp, hanging over my arms, pupils fixed and unresponsive, glaring into nothingness.

Oh my God ... OH MY GOD ... my mind went into overload. She just died right here in my arms, this cannot be, this is not possible, she cannot be dead, not now.

"Honey ... HONEY ..." I tried to get a response.

The inside of my whole body trembled, my arms and shoulders were shaking, fear rapidly took over, my heart pounded in my throat and drummed in my ears.

"BECKY ... BECKY," with a louder, but clearly fear-filled voice.

Slowly I twisted my body so I was able to lower hers gently onto the ground, alongside the bathtub. Her body still lifeless, her eyes still wide open, not responding, gazing into nowhere. As I gently advanced to ease her body onto the ground, her hands were the first to arrive onto the floor, still no response. Her head in my left hand, her motionless body supported by my right. No breathing detectable, her chest motionless.

"Becky ...BECKY ..." louder but now with a distinct purpose.

I was trying to arouse her. My right hand now on her shoulder, I softly shook her. Instinctively I checked for a pulse. I placed my index finger and middle finger, side by side, in her neck, trying to find a pulsating movement from her carotid artery. Nothing.

I need to start CPR now! I was thinking. *This cannot be happening.*

Connor's voice, filled with worry, came from the living room.

"Papa, are you ok?"

My brain was in a haze. His voice in the distance, faded. I did not register, everything was muffled...sounds, vision, feelings.

"Papa...?" Connor once again asked.

His voice penetrated through the air and reached me with accurate precision. It awoke me from my trance and sounds reappeared. Now fully alert,

"Connor," I responded, "grab the phone from the kitchen and call 911!"

Although he was unaware of what was happening, he understood, and without hesitation he knew what he had to do. With his small hand holding the cordless phone pressed to his face, he appeared in the doorway. He stood there staring at me with his eyes screaming fear and confusion. Within seconds, Dane stepped right next to him. His eyes aimed at his mama, then with his eyes filled with questions and fear he stared at me.

My attention focused on them, it tore me apart to see those two sweet boys standing there alone in the hallway, staring at their mama, not knowing what was going on, not knowing what happened, but too scared to ask.

The picture they were seeing, where their papa was sitting on the ground, holding the lifeless body of their mama, was evidence of a situation they had been fearing. The silence was loud, the air heavy, the sadness around us was suffocating.

"Is mama...?" Connor asked.

The fear for what he had been pushing away, deep inside him, came to the surface.

As I was preparing myself to speak the most difficult words a parent could ever say to a child, I felt a sudden, soft movement in my arms. Abruptly I aborted the formulation of my answer to Connor. Becky's eyes regained focus, her pupils now aimed at me, slowly life came back into her body. Her chest gently began to rise and fall, and her left hand lifted up to touch my face. Although all my attention was directed to Becky, I responded to Connor's question,

"No, sweetie, mama is ok. She just passed out."

My soul inside jumped, joy was overwhelming my fear and pushed it aside. She raised her hand and gently stroked it along my cheek. Her voice silent, her eyes loving and tender. My lips quivered, with a broken voice, I tried to comfort her.

"You're ok baby, you're ok."

She smiled.

She never knew, I never told her. Connor or Dane never knew, I never told them either. I thought that at this moment I had lost her. It was a secret locket inside me, but this ferocious event left a deep and irreparable scar on my soul.

Dane's face unfolded in a smile when he saw his mama responding. His eyes glittered from joy. Connor's fearful gaze was replaced with a soft but noticeable sigh. He was still holding on to the phone, it never left the side of his face as he continued to update the 911-dispatcher about what was going on. The suffocating air became lighter and breathable for us all.

I cannot imagine what was going through their little minds, but the fear in their eyes told a painful and worrisome story. Their motionless pose, like statues, at the bathroom door with both of them absorbing the horrific display of their mama being held in the arms of their Papa, illustrated the brutal terror that kept their young souls hostage.

They were too young to be here, to be in this situation. It was unfair that this was happening to them. As a father I wanted to protect them, shield them from this pain, wrap my arms around them, hold them close to me and have all of us wake up from this gruesome nightmare.

Lisa arrived at our home before the ambulance did. When you are a firefighter, those things tend to happen since most of us would be listening to the scanner, even if you are not on duty that night. I am sure that Lisa recognized the address when the 911-call from Connor tripped the fire department for assistance.

I was still on the floor in the bathroom with Becky in my arms, who was now slowly getting more and more alert. The boys were still standing motionless in the hallway, watching us. I could hear the front door being opened in a more than usual rough manner. The little doorbells that were attached to the inside doorknob, to alert us for when someone was coming in, made a louder and more distinct sound than usual.

Immediately Lisa announced her arrival.

"It is just me guys! Where are you at?"

Followed by rapid footsteps up the stairs. Within seconds she was standing behind Connor and Dane, looking at me with eyes filled with questions. But before she could say anything, I enlightened her by answering her question.

"She just passed out," I said.

Becky turned her head to get a glimpse of the person to whom I was talking to.

"Hey, Lisa," she nonchalantly stated, as if nothing had happened.

Although I displayed confidence and brushed the whole incident off as 'a syncopal episode', on the inside I was still screaming out loud, my soul trembling from fear, still trying to recover from the instilled despair that I had just experienced; the loss of my love, then her sudden return.

From my position on the floor, I was able to see across the hallway into the boys' bedroom. The door was open, and the windows were positioned right above the garage, facing the driveway. While I talked to Lisa, from the corner of my eye I saw a blue and red reflection bouncing off the bedroom wall. My eyes deviated just a miniscule fraction from my conversation with Lisa, but apparently enough for her to realize that my attention was pulled away for something that was happening behind her. She glanced over her shoulder to observe the same red and blue reflection, now brightly bursting through the windows. "

Ah, the boys are here," she said.

All firefighters from our department were also medics. Some were EMTs, others were Paramedics. Most of them had been to our home as friends and celebrated many birthdays with us. Lisa walked back to the front door to let them in. From the chatter, I recognized their voices. While they were making their way up to us, Becky looked at me with anxious eyes.

"I think I am fine honey," she said.

I took a deep breath in and exhaled and tipped my head to the right.

"I know babe, but it is important to get this checked out tonight, ok?" I responded.

Her immediate cooperation and willingness to go to the ER was a strong indication that she was also concerned. Her voice remained silent, but her eyes unfolded the truth. The excruciating pain in her chest that led to the actual loss of consciousness, the fear for the uncontrollable was very real. It did not back up and it could return at any moment, at any time, without warning or regret.

It was good to see that both medics were friends. It always makes these already stressful situations a little easier, especially for Connor and Dane. They were both still in shock about what had just happened. I am sure they were wondering what was going to happen next. Seeing paramedics arriving in an ambulance was scary enough. It made it a little easier when they recognized those that would be taking away their mama.

The space between the cabinets and bathtub was fairly small. Becky was lying completely stretched out, but I was folded up awkwardly with my legs twisted against the tub and my back pressed onto the cabinets with one handle poking painfully into my shoulder blade. The paramedics placed the cot in the hallway, close to the bathroom door against the wall. As they came in, they explained that they would help Becky get from there to the cot. The tallest one stepped over our bodies and squatted next to us on the right, while the other stood on the left of us.

"Roy, I will support her head, I want you to get out of there," he said, "It looks really uncomfortable," with a big smile on his face.

As he placed both his hands under Becky's shoulders, using his forearms to support her head, I wiggled myself from underneath Becky. My left hand reached over my head and grabbed the edge of the counter while the other one was finding support on the edge of the bathtub in front of me. My knees were stiff and unwilling to stretch completely. Once I stood up, I stepped sideways to allow them as much space as possible. I reached the bathroom door without any hiccups. I wrapped both boys in my arms, kissed them and squeezed their bodies against mine.

"You guys ok?" I asked, concerned.

Becky was standing in the middle of the bathroom, bathtub behind her, counter in front of her. The paramedic on her left had placed his arm underneath hers, the other paramedic on the right, stepping backwards giving instructions, telling her what to do.

"Follow me Becky," he said.

As she turned to follow him out of the bathroom, she placed both her hands in his for support. The other paramedic wrapped his hands around her torso for extra assistance. With little baby-steps, inch by inch, she stepped forward closer to the cot in the hallway.

"I can do this ... I can do this," Becky said to encourage herself.

As she moved through the bathroom with her two supporters, like a couple of bookends providing stability, both Connor and Dane were awfully quiet. Their silence, their posture, their motionless stance, explained that they were very troubled by this event.

Becky made it to the cot, and both paramedics were working on getting her comfortable. Before I left for the hospital, I knew I had to talk to my boys. I kneeled right in front of them and leaned my back against the wall for support, my eyes aimed at them.

"Ok guys" I said, "we need to know why this happened to mama tonight, so we are going to the hospital to figure it out, ok?"

Their little heads nodded; their eyes sad.

"Are you staying at the hospital again tonight?" Dane asked with a slight quiver in his voice, revealing the misery he was in.

I understood all too well the fear they were consistently facing. I knew they tried to push it away as much as possible, but during these moments, when their mama was being strapped to a cot and taken away by ambulance, it must have been one of their most frightening ones. My response, as always, was nothing less than the truth.

"I don't know sweetie. It depends on what they figure out tonight."

The hospital room was dark, and silence had taken over. The dim muteness provided for an unnatural, yet comfortable calmness. The digital clock on the nightstand to the left of Becky announced that it was 3:14 AM. Becky had been asleep for hours.

We arrived at the hospital after an uneventful ambulance ride. Once in the ER, Becky had several additional episodes of severe pain and received numerous doses of morphine to control it. Multiple tests were completed: EKG, chest X-ray, and blood work, but nothing revealed anything abnormal that was causing these chest pains. The ER doctor determined that it was better for Becky to stay in the hospital that night.

"Here we can control your pain better," he explained, "and I am scheduling you for an esophageal scope tomorrow morning."

My eyes were blank, staring at Becky's silhouette. My brain was working overtime, trying to make sense of it all. Revisiting the moments in the bathroom when Becky had stood up and started to stumble my way, her eyes clawed into me with a desperate scream for help. When she collapsed in my arms, with her eyes wide open, her body limp, for a moment I thought she died right there in my arms. God, what a horrible feeling.

The heaviness of the day was wearing me down, my soul tired, my strength tested. The blackness of the room instilled some peace, causing my mind to wander back to past times when life was less complicated. Back to that time I took Becky to the Netherlands for the first time: It was in October 1998.

It was a long flight to Amsterdam. We arrived at Schiphol Airport early in the morning, around eight am. Once we cleared customs, we walked through the hallway on the left that was marked with a large green sign that stated, "NOTHING TO DECLARE." The hallway on the right had a large red sign that stated, "SOMETHING TO DECLARE." Personally, I always believed that if they made these signs in a neutral color, more people might be honest and go through the 'something to declare' side. A big red sign just warrants avoidance.

My parents were waiting for us at the other side of the sliding doors. It was thrilling for me to see my parents again, and it was exciting for Becky to finally meet them. After a couple cups of coffee at a small café in the airport, trying to regain energy from the long flight and time difference, we left for my parents' home where we would be staying for the next nine days. The attic room was a large bedroom with a small couch, coffee table and TV, almost like a studio.

Since it is seven hours later in the Netherlands, the jet lag is brutal for the first two to three days. You could be in the middle of a conversation at one moment, and two minutes later you would be knocked out for a thirty-minute nap. At the weirdest times you ended up taking naps, but after those first rough days, your body eventually adjusts.

I remember on the fourth night we decided to go out for dinner to give my mother a break from cooking meals. We went to a nice restaurant called *'De Driesprong'* (means the 'T-intersection'), located at the 'Loosdrechtse Plassen' (this literally means, 'the lakes at Loosdrecht', which is a small town close to where my parents lived). We had great food and some nice red wine. The view from the restaurant was breathtaking; right on the lakes with the sun sinking into the trees at the far end, reflecting onto the water.

When we got back to my parents' house, Becky wanted to go straight to bed. The good food and wine made her sleepier. I stayed with my parent's downstairs just a little longer to share some more time with them.

It was nice to talk to my parents face-to-face for a change. Normally my father would call me every Sunday to chit chat. Sometimes we would spend only five minutes on the phone, sometimes we talked for an hour, but it was always good to talk to them.

My dad was an old military guy. He joined the navy at an early age right after WWII, spending most of his time in the military. Always away from home on a ship somewhere on the planet, for many months he would be gone. It made him stubborn, he was always right, and not much of a communicator.

A massive heart attack in January 1992 shook his world and changed his perspective on life. He became more appreciative of the little things, such as spending more time with his sons. He became more of a hugger, but still he would never say 'I love you.' In his mind that was a given fact.

"You are my son, of course I love you, I don't have to say that," would be his response.

My dad was sitting in 'his' chair. It was a light brown leather, perfectly positioned straight in front of the TV, with his own side-table made of old worn oak with a smaller lower shelf for magazines. On the other side of the chair was a standing light-fixture to provide him, and only him, or whomever was sitting in his chair if he was not home, with illumination.

Tonight was no different than any night at my parents' home. My mom would make sure that everyone had something to drink, then snacks would be placed on the coffee table that was standing in front of the love seat. These snacks would be typical Dutch, ranging from 'kroketten' and 'bitterballen' to small squares of cheese. The TV would be on, but with low volume to provide some background noise.

My dad was sitting in his chair, sipping on some red wine. He would lean forward now and then to retrieve a little snack from the wood cutting board my mother used as a serving tray.

My mom was standing in the kitchen at the counter. In front of her were more 'bitterballen' on a small metal tray, ready to be warmed up in the oven. She looked at me and asked,

"What do you want to drink, sweetie?"

As usual, I would drink 'Jonge Genever' (a Dutch gin) mixed with diet Coke. I planted myself on the right side of the love seat, closest to my dad. With my mom still standing in the kitchen, we all talked about dinner and how impressed we were with the quality of the food and service.

My dad was staring at me, and from the look of his eyes I could see he was mauling his brain inside to determine the proper words to choose for the next sentence that would leave his lips. He placed his left arm on the armrest of the chair, leaned towards me, raised his right hand, pointed his finger at me, indicating that he was going to say something important. He looked me straight in the eyes when his words came straight from his heart,

"She is a good girl."

The gaze from his eyes did not deter, his face still with the same expression, his finger still in the air. He continued his mission about his vision,

"She has a good and kind heart."

He was dead serious, he never ever said that to me about anyone. His words arrived with chilling precision into my heart. I stood up, walked over to him, put my arms around his neck, placed my lips on his cheek to confirm my love for him and whispered softly,

"I know Papa."

He accepted that as the proper answer for the statements he made. It was a well-kept secret between us, since he never spoke about that again, not to me, not to Becky or anyone. I knew, he knew, and that was all that mattered.

Eleven

The air-conditioning was blowing full force. The cold draft coming from above rushing over our skin caused chills and goosebumps. Normally I enjoy the cooler environment, but today it just felt too frigid. Maybe it was the lack of sleep, maybe the lack of proper nutrition, or maybe the increased stress. Becky was huddling under her blanket, trying to shield herself from this cold arctic blast. I tucked the blanket around her like a burrito, so that only her face was showing. Yesterday, the ER doctor ordered an esophageal scope to rule out any abnormalities of the esophagus or stomach. He was able to get us in for this EGD (*EsophagoGastroDuodenoscopy)* first thing in the morning.

It was barely 6 AM, and the pre-procedure room had a total of eight beds, four at each side. They were all perfectly made; the creme colored blankets, flawlessly tucked around the mattress. The white sheet underneath the blanket was folded around the top near the pillow, causing a white banner. All the beds were exactly the same, produced with military precision.

At the foot-end of all beds lay an impeccable folded blue hospital gown, topped with a blue see-through surgical hoody and a pair of grey hospital socks with white rubber enhancements on both sides of the feet to prevent slipping on the slick hospital floors.

On the walls behind each bed sat a large suction device with hoses and a monitor to display heart rate, blood pressure, and oxygen saturation. The blood-pressure cuff, the four EKG lead wiring, and the pulse-oximetry device that slides on the finger, were all conveniently placed in a small wire basket below the monitor. Every bed was separated by a curtain that could be pulled around each bed. At that time, all curtains were still pulled back to the walls since there was no one in this area but us.

Once the nurse completed all her required assessments, she explained that both the anesthesiologist and the specialist would soon stop by.

"We never know who stops by first," she said, "but they will be here shortly."

She closed the curtain around us, just to provide us with a little more privacy.

I moved my chair closer to Becky's bed, placed my hand on her leg that was now covered with three warm blankets.

"How is your chest pain babe?" I asked, while my hand made gentle short strokes on her leg.

"Doing better," she answered. "It was so painful and I was so scared."

The fear appeared back into her eyes.

"I know babe," I said.

I never told her that I thought she died right there in my arms. I never explained to her how mortified I was when I stood there holding her lifeless body. I never shared that with her. I did not want her to worry about me, she had enough to worry about. I did not want her to be concerned about my wellbeing, and although I never said anything, I think she knew.

The anesthesiologist asked the obvious standard questions about allergies and if Becky ever had any adverse reactions or complications during previous surgeries. After he left, he closed the curtain behind him, but within five minutes another gentleman appeared.

He stood still in front of the curtains and announced his arrival by saying,

"Knock, knock, ... anyone home?"

"Come on in, the door is open," Becky said with a big smile on her face.

A tall man appeared. He had dark brown curly hair with some grey spots here and there. He was normal built and had a soft deep voice. While he completed his detailed assessment, he asked questions about the chest pain episodes from yesterday.

Suddenly Becky stopped him, and with a sparkle of menace in her eyes and joy on her face, she said,

"Do you know that you look like Jimmy Buffet?"

He tilted his head to the left, pouted his lips, placed his left hand on his chin, and as his finger stroked his jaw line,

"Well, I have to say that's the first time someone has told me that," he said with a big smile, "but I like his music, does that count?"

Becky laughed out loud, her eyes cheerfully glowing, and a big wide smile on her face,

"Well, you have to know that I am a real parrot-head, and I am telling everyone that Jimmy Buffet did surgery on me today."

A frown appeared as he raised his left eyebrow, and the puzzled look in his eyes explained that he was unaware of the term 'parrot-head'.

Becky noticed his confusion and informed him that the term 'parrot-head' is used for those who are true Jimmy Buffet fans.

"Ah," he chanted, "well, I am not doing surgery on you today, just taking a look down there," as he placed his hand on her foot.

"I will see you shortly," he said as he disappeared through the curtains.

Becky, smiling, sat straight up in bed.

"Don't you think he looks like Jimmy?" she asked.

I did see some resemblance, but he was not like his twin brother. While we were talking about this Jimmy Buffet look-alike doctor the nurse opened the curtains and explained that they were ready. I walked along with them, right next to Becky's bed, holding her hand. The nurse navigated the bed with accurate precision around the corners and through multiple doors, then she stopped.

"We have to go in here, time to let go" she said smiling.

I leaned forward, and as we hugged, our lips touched, our eyes closed, and our souls connected. Another moment where we were forced to let go of each other. Another moment where we were separated. Another moment where we had to worry about what they would discover. It is not just another test, but another confirmation of the inevitable realization of how sick Becky truly was, and how ruthless cancer can be.

Becky's eyes told her unspoken fear, the worries, the pain, the 'I don't want to be here.' All I could do was to be there for her, support her, no matter what or how. As our lips slowly let go, I placed my forehead against hers, and as my left hand gently stroked her cheekbone, I said,

"I love you babe. I will be right here waiting for you. Don't worry, everything will be fine."

The nurse opened the doors to the procedure area with the large red knob on the wall right next to us, then she pushed Becky through the opening. Our eyes did not let go until she turned around the corner, and right before Becky disappeared from my view, she lifted her hand from the bed, touched her lips with her fingers, and blew a kiss.

Every time I saw her being pushed off to some kind of test or procedure, it hurt. Too many times I sat there, alone, waiting for her to come back out.

On my way back to the waiting area, I just wondered why her … why not me … why …?

We got back to Becky's room, on 8-south, just past lunchtime. The bed in her room had clean sheets and blankets folded around the mattress with the same military style precision we saw earlier in the procedure room. The room was clean, trash removed, and floor mopped. You could still smell the odor of the fresh orange scent from the cleaner they used. The sun was high in the sky, beaming through the window leaving short shadows on the ground. The air-conditioning was working overtime, blowing cooled air softly into the room, causing the cream-colored curtains to dance delicately.

The floor nurse appeared right after she noticed that we were back in Becky's room. Even though the door was wide open, she alerted us of her arrival by knocking on the door post. Becky and I were pleased to see it was one of our favorite nurses on this floor. Before she started working here on 8-south, the oncology floor, she used to work in the ER with me. The first time Becky was admitted to this floor, she was our nurse and immediately there was a connection.

She stepped into the room with a big smile on her face and bright eyed.

"Hey guys!" she exclaimed, "Not happy to see you here, but happy to be your nurse."

Becky immediately opened up her arms to welcome her. After hugs and hello's, she explained that Doctor Freeman stopped by during his early morning rounds, but since we were not here, he would stop by around five this afternoon.

"How did the scope go this morning?" she asked.

Becky explained, while giggling, that the GI-specialist looked like Jimmy Buffet, but that the procedure went well. No results yet, but everything seemed to look normal besides a small blister of some sorts that was found in her esophagus.

The shadows on the floor were stretching longer as the sun started towards the west horizon. My lower back was stiff from the uncomfortable position in the recliner. I fell asleep while Becky was taking a nap after she had some lunch. I looked over to my left, to where Becky's bed was. She did not notice that I had woken up. The head of her bed almost upright, her reading glasses on the tip of her nose, magnifying the words in her book she was reading. Fixated on the story, she was sitting motionless, besides the page flipping action.

"How are you doing babe?" I asked.

She turned her head in my direction, keeping the book in the same position and smiled,

"Okay, I guess ..." she said, "... I can feel some more pain again in my chest."

That was not something I wanted to hear, but before I could answer, there were two loud knocks on the door.

"It is Doctor Freeman," he announced as he stepped into the room.

His appearance always brought some joy to both Becky and me. His kind face, perky eyes, pleasant smile, and soft considerate voice was comforting. As always, he was very proper in his approach, shaking hands and asking how we were doing. He explained that he just had a conversation with the GI-specialist, the Jimmy Buffet look-alike, about the procedure from this morning. He took a sample of the blister-like tissue, and we would get results within a week or so.

While walking towards the side of the bed, he pulled out his stethoscope from the pocket of his jacket, and started to unfold it without looking at it, as if he had done that a million times. He asked Becky to lean forward so he could listen to her lungs. Becky sat up straight, her hands forward along her legs to support herself. Doctor Freeman placed the stethoscope on the middle section of her back. After he completed the auscultation of her lungs, he placed the stethoscope back into his pocket.

"Tell me about the chest pain you had Becky." he asked.

"Well," Becky started, "funny you should ask, because I think I have one coming on right now!"

Her eyes shooting looks of fear, arching her back, as she started to tap furiously on her chest with her right hand. Her face pale, her eyes seeking for relief.

"It hurts... it hurts..."

Doctor Freeman reached out his right hand, passed Becky, towards the red button on the wall right behind her. He activated the emergency button and within seconds a female voice responded,

"How may I assist you?"

Doctor Freeman's demeanor had changed to a man on a mission, he was all business. His eyes focused on Becky, he had only one goal; taking care of her, his patient, taking away that pain. With a direct and strong voice, he provided the person on the other side of the line with clear orders,

"This is Doctor Freeman. I need two milligrams of IV morphine into room 814 STAT!"

Becky was in obvious pain and severe distress, her breathing rapid and shallow, almost panting, the knuckles of her hand white, bald fist pounding on her chest trying to relieve the pain, eyes staring straight ahead.

"It hurts...it hurts..."

I was standing on the right side of the bed, with my hand placed on her leg. Doctor Freeman stood on the other side, trying to calm her by coaching her through the pain. She looked at me and her eyes screamed for help, she was spiraling down fast. The floor nurse arrived with a rapid stride through the door. Her eyes were flying around the room, assessing the situation in a split second. Armed with a syringe, filled with the two milligrams of morphine as ordered, she walked over to the IV tubing hanging right behind Becky.

Doctor Freeman confirmed,

"Administer two of morphine please."

The nurse injected the medicine through the medication port, just half-way down the IV-tubing, and flushed it into Becky's system with a normal saline flush. She confirmed,

"Two of morphine given..." quickly glancing at her watch "... at 18:10."

Becky continued to tap her chest like a drum,

"Nothing is happening...nothing is happening!"

Doctor Freeman seemed to be waiting for improvement. After several minutes he assured himself that there was no relief and placed another order with the nurse,

"Please get four more of morphine."

As the nurse walked away to get the additional medication, she confirmed the order,

"Four more of morphine."

Doctor Freeman placed his hand on Becky's shoulder and explained,

"This is probably going to knock you out, but I don't want you to be in any pain."

Becky stared at him with a solid and determined look,

"I don't care what you have to do, but stop this pain!"

The nurse returned with the additional morphine. Right before she was ready to administer it, she re-confirmed with Freeman,

"Four more of morphine?"

"Yes please, four more of morphine," Freeman stated, determined to eliminate Becky's pain.

After the medication was released into the IV-tubing, she flushed it once again with a normal saline flush. Although morphine is clear, you could actually see the medicine flowing down the IV tubing. It causes a distortion of the clear fluid.

Within seconds it reached the port under Becky's skin, to be released into her body. Almost instantly there was a noticeable difference in Becky's behavior; the rapid tapping on her chest became slower and slower, her reflexes decreased, her arms started to sink lower. Gradually her breathing decreased into a relaxing rhythm. She lowered her torso on the bed and landed gently on the mattress.

"Don't worry," Doctor Freeman said, "it is just the morphine. It knocked her out."

As Becky's eyes slowly closed, he continued,

"I was hoping that two milligrams of morphine would take care of it, but this seems to be an intense pain."

Becky's breathing was slow and calm.

"I can see why she had a syncopal episode with this severity at home."

He looked at the floor nurse and ordered a PCA-pump, (Patient Controlled Analgesia) with morphine for pain control.

A PCA-pump is a device that is attached to the IV-line. Inside the pump is a large unit of pain mediation, such as morphine, that can be administered by the patient self by pushing on a button. There are maximums to the amount of medication that can be given. Normally the patient can push the button for pain control every 5 or 10 minutes.

Doctor Freeman looked at me and stuck his hand straight out to shake mine. His eyes never looked away, his grip firm, determined, but gentle.

"I will be back tomorrow morning with morning rounds," he said, "I will put in a standing order for additional morphine in her chart in case she has another pain attack."

He slowly released his grip.

"I want her to stay here for a couple of days so we can get that pain under control, okay?" he said.

We both nodded at the same time.

"Okay," I responded, to confirm his plan.

The sun started to break through the horizon, pushing the darkness of the night out of view. The days were getting shorter and the nights longer, the arrival of fall was upon us. This was the fifth morning here on 8-south, the oncology floor. Over the last several days, the boys had been taken care of by Lisa and family members. I went home several times to be with the boys, and to try to accomplish a normal routine for them. When I was home, a friend or family member would stay with Becky overnight at the hospital.

Being home at night allowed me to spend some time with Connor and Dane, sleep at home, have a shower, wake up with them in the morning, make them some breakfast, and take them to school.

Those were difficult times. As a husband you want to be where your wife is, but as a father you want to be there for your kids. So, the only way to accomplish a little of both, was by travelling between locations, having short nights, and skipping meals. I tried my best to keep things as normal as possible for Connor and Dane.

Last night though, I just wanted to be with Becky, be with my wife, kiss her lips goodnight, sleep close to her. Lisa offered to spend the night with the boys, and she took them to school in the morning. Becky's chest-pain attacks had slowly diminished in frequency and intensity. Yesterday she only used the PCA-pump once, and based on that, she would be discharged soon.

I was sitting in the recliner, staring outside the window. My left hand placed on Becky's leg, observing the start of another day. The tray-table was in front of Becky, she was sitting upright, with the back of the bed in the most upright position. The green plastic plate cover, to keep the food hot, was laying on the far-left corner of the table, Becky was trying to eat some grits with honey. It was always one of her favorites, but she had not been eating well ever since she became ill. She had lost a lot of weight over the last several months. At one point she was losing so much that Doctor Freeman told her that she had to start eating more, or he would stop the medication for the cancer treatment.

"What good is it if, on one hand you are taking medication to fight the cancer, but on the other hand you are starving to death," he told her during a clinic visit.

A very true statement. I knew Becky was trying to eat better, but I also understood that she just did not have much of an appetite. I tried my best to provide her with healthy foods with high nutritional value, all fresh, all made from scratch, no preservatives, all organic, and no GMOs. Regardless of my efforts, she continued to lose weight.

She had only taken a couple of bites of her grits this morning and pushed the table to the side.

"I will eat the rest later," she said.

I lowered the head of the bed for her comfort. I sat down next to her when she grabbed my hand.

"Honey," she said as she stared at me with those intense black round holes surrounded by clear bright emerald green.

A slight tremble in her voice revealed that she was concerned and serious. Her right hand had a hold of my left, her grip weak but strong enough to hold me in place. Her movements were slow but deliberate and determined, her left hand moved closer, something was inside her palm, undetectable to the eye, well hidden from sight.

As her hand moved closer to mine, her fingers unfolded the truth and carefully she slid her wedding-band onto my pinky finger. A perfect fit, as if it was specially made for it. My eyes told her that I was confused and not liking the situation. Her dried cracked lips released the painful truth.

"It keeps falling off honey," she said.

"Please wear it for me, I will put it back on when I start gaining some more weight, okay?"

As these words escaped from her mouth, we both had the realization that from now on this was the last time she would display to the world her status as a married woman.

Silence filled the room with an intense weight. Our eyes connected, yet nothing was said. The sadness was intense, but she knew that I would wear her ring with honor and pride.

Twelve

The exam room at Doctor Freeman's office was, as usual, spotlessly clean. Only the necessary items were purposefully placed at particular areas. The desk was plain and clear of clutter. There was a computer screen, keyboard, and a notepad, hugged by a writing instrument. It has been almost a month since we had seen Doctor Freeman. It has been three months since the initial diagnosis of stage IV non-small cell lung cancer.

Today was the day that we would see if we were on the right track; to confirm that what we were doing was the right approach. We attacked the cancer from two sides, a holistic and conventional method. We tried to defeat it with not only medicine, but also with a massive shift in diet, juicing, and the use of glyconutrients. Although there were many bumps on the road over the last three months, today we would get the results from the PET-scan that was completed two days ago.

Becky seemed to be doing a little better. She had more energy, tried to maintain weight, and her eye was almost back to normal. We were sitting next to each other, holding hands, patiently waiting for Doctor Freeman to deliver the results. A soft knock on the door announced his arrival. He walked in with his usual addictive smile. He was always proper and positive, no matter how bad things were. He never sugar-coated anything and was always straightforward and direct, putting everything on the table, good or bad.

After his assessment of how Becky was doing and feeling, he went into details about the latest PET-scan. He opened a program on his computer and the screen displayed many images. He invited us to come closer. I moved a chair right next to Freeman's chair and helped Becky to sit down in it. She was now facing the screen straight on. I stood behind her and placed my hands on her shoulders. Her right hand moved up to grab my left hand. Doctor Freeman opened the program and placed the pictures of two different PET-scans next to each other. His index finger pointed at the left one.

"This was your initial scan in July," he said.

His finger glided over the screen until he pointed at the right one.

"And this one is from two days ago."

He circled the bright reddened areas on both pictures on the screen.

"As you can see, the new scan shows a decrease in size of the tumor in your left lung," he said with a delicate smile on his face.

"It went down from about four centimeters in diameter to two-and-a-half!"

Becky's hand squeezed mine, shaking from excitement, she yelled,

"Yay!"

I felt relief, a massive block of concrete just fell off my shoulders.

It is working! I thought.

It was positive news for a change. It seemed that all the things we were doing actually helped, almost a 50% decrease in size.

Doctor Freeman was 'carefully' optimistic and advised us to continue with whatever we were doing. It was a good day. It was an unexpected arrival of positive news. I know we were both hoping for a positive development. The last three months had been an emotional rollercoaster, but now it seemed that we were on the right track. Becky's eyes sparkled so bright she lit up the room. I could feel her soul jumping up and down from excitement.

***

Becky was up early. Even though she was staying in bed, it was nice to have her awake while I was getting the boys ready for school. I made breakfast burritos and the house was filled with the scent of fried eggs, cheese and turkey. Despite the wonderful mixture of aromas, Becky just wanted tea with honey and some oatmeal. The boys were sitting at the dining room table, eating and talking about some video game they had been playing.

I poured the hot water in a large mug on top of the teabag that danced with the water. As the teabag slowly began to absorb the hot liquid, the dancing slowed down and it started to sink to the bottom of the mug. A tablespoon filled with organic local honey came down into the water to be mixed into a dark amber beverage. I placed the tea with the oatmeal on the bed-tray and walked it carefully over to our bedroom. Becky was reading in bed.

"Breakfast is served Ma'am," I jokingly announced when I walked in.

She smiled, took her glasses off, placed the book next to her, open with the pages down,

"Thank you honey," she said.

She folded her hands around the mug, and right before she placed her lips on the rim, she pouted them and gently blew a delicate breeze over the hot surface causing a soft detour of the steam away from her face. After a small sip, she placed the mug back on the tray, and placed both of her warmed hands in the nape of her neck, softly rubbing it.

"My neck is really hurting," she said, as she twisted her neck to the left trying to relieve the pain.

Over the last several weeks, she had been complaining about neck pain numerous times, but this week it seemed to happen more often and with greater intensity. At times it was so bad that I had to give her muscle relaxers and narcotic painkillers to ease the pain.

The problem with those painkillers was that they would help, but it also knocked her out. She would sleep for hours, and that would cause her to skip doses of her Tarceva. We both thought it was just neck pain from stress, but it was becoming more concerning.

I always tried to be as quiet as possible upon entering the house, because I never knew if Becky was asleep or not. Today was no different. After I dropped Connor and Dane off at school, I carefully opened the front door, trying not to disturb the little bell that was hanging on the inside on the door lever. When I got to the landing on top of the stairs, between the living room and the hallway, I could hear Becky moan. Softly and distant, but it traveled from our bedroom through the hallway, at regular intervals. I made my way to our bedroom and the sound of weeping increased. Becky was curled up in a fetal position, her hands around her neck, her shoulder shrugging, tears falling from her eyes, her body softly rocking back and forth.

"Oh honey," she said with a shaky voice, "it is so bad right now."

I squatted right next to the bed, placed my hand on the side of her neck, gently stroking it, as if I were trying to rub the pain away. I hated to see her in so much agony. My heart was falling into a thousand little pieces. It was tearing me apart to see how my sweetheart was being demolished by this brutal and heartless disease. As I wiped away her tears with my thumb, I said,

"I am calling Doctor Freeman babe; this is getting out of control."

Her silence proved agreement.

A kind female voice answered the call, "Mercy Cancer Center. How may I assist you?"

"This is Roy Slootheer," I said, "can I talk to Doctor Freeman or his nurse Angie please."

"One moment," the lady explained on the other side, "let me page them for you."

Within a minute Angie answered, "Hey Roy, what's going on?"

I explained in detail how Becky's neck pain was getting to a point that was unbearable for her.

"Let me talk to Doctor Freeman," Angie said, "I will be right back."

While I was on hold, I sat down next to Becky on the bed, stroking her hair, trying to comfort her. I already gave her some Norco (an opioid painkiller), but she did not like that much because it made her loopy, but it was better than dealing with that pain.

Doctor Freeman came on the phone. "What is happening Roy?" he asked me.

We discussed the situation in detail. He was aware of the intermittent neck pain and stiffness over the last several weeks, and that Becky was taking a lot of pain killers to deal with it.

"Can you take her to the hospital?" he asked.

"I want to admit her for pain control and to do some additional testing."

"We are on my way," I said.

Becky was curled up in the car seat, her left shoulder raised up towards her neck, as if it were releasing some of the pain. Her lips pushed together, almost in a straight line. Her eyebrows molted into a frown, her eyes staring at the dashboard of my truck. Regardless of the painkillers I gave her, she continued to be in a lot of misery. I tried to get to the hospital as fast as I could. The faster I got there, the sooner she would be able to get some relief from the IV medication. I parked the truck in front of the main entrance.

"I will be right back sweetie," I explained. "I am going to get you a wheelchair."

There were always wheelchairs placed by the front entrance inside the hospital. I stepped through the large rotating doors and grabbed one. I placed it alongside the truck, on the passenger side, opened Becky's door and helped her to get out. Although she was still in pain, she managed to smile at me as she sat down in the wheelchair.

The gentleman at the check-in counter tried to speed up the admission process as much as he could. He saw that Becky was in a lot of pain. I informed him that Becky was a 'direct admit' from Doctor Freeman. After we answered some standard questions, he said,

"I have you right here in the system, you will be going to room 825."

He pushed several keys on the keyboard and the printer that was positioned right behind him made a soft buzzing sound. He removed the sheet of paper from the tray, flipped it over and checked the information. He removed an elongated self-adhesive strip from the top part of the paper and folded it around Becky's wrist.

"You guys are all good to go," he confirmed.

We passed the nurse's station on the 8th floor. I slowed down my pace, but never stopped. I informed the receptionist of our arrival.

"We are here for room 825."

She leaned over to check Becky's bracelet and after she confirmed, she instructed us to go ahead to the room.

"The nurse will be right there," she said.

As I pushed the wheelchair through the hallway, a female voice came on the intercom and announced,

"New admit for room 825 has arrived."

The door to the room was wide open, the window showed little specks of water from the rain that had just started. These hospital rooms were becoming too familiar, the people working on this floor were getting too common and knowing our way around was not something to be joyful about. We rolled into this chamber of depression where pain and misery lived. Another visit to the hospital was not on our to-do list, but yet, here we were again.

I helped Becky out of the wheelchair up to the edge of the bed. She sat down to put on the depression-blue hospital gown. Suddenly the floodgates opened. Tears poured down her cheeks like waterfalls, her shoulders quivering, gently moving up and down in sync with the soft sobbing sounds escaping from her lips. Regardless if it was because of the continuous uncontrollable pain in her neck, or because we were back in the hospital again, I wrapped her in my arms, and pulled her close. She placed her head against my chest. The quiver from inside her soul contagiously took a hold of mine. Although I was trying to stand strong, I was unable to resist. My eyes swelled up and released a delicate flow of tears filled with pain, slowly running down my face. We just sat there, as one, silently. Our souls as one, our hearts bleeding together.

The lights inside the MRI room were dimmed. Prior to our arrival, the nurse administered some Ativan via Becky's port to calm her. Becky always had been claustrophobic, and these MRI machines were small long tubes that would scare most people. The Ativan would help her to calm down enough to go through the procedure.

Since an MRI is a large magnet, no one but the patient was allowed in the procedure room.

Becky was laying on a small skinny table that would disappear into this tube. I did not know if she was shivering because she was cold, or because she was scared, but the technician was so nice to bring her some warm blankets. I helped him place these over Becky, tucking the edges underneath her. She seemed just a little more comfortable. I kissed her soft lips.

"I will be waiting outside honey, " I told her.

Her eyes were filled with fear. She did not like this, she hated small spaces, and this MRI machine was too small for comfort. As the technician walked out with me, the large door closed behind us.

"It will take about 40 minutes to complete," he informed me.

"If you want to, you can go to the waiting area and get some coffee. I will come and get you as soon as she is ready."

The waiting room had about four people spread throughout the area. The TV was on but the sound was turned down. A large coffee machine was standing along the far end wall. It was one of those fancy devices that could make all kinds of beverages from regular coffee, to hot chocolate, to a vanilla latte.

I stood right in front of it and the smell of fresh coffee with a hint of sweetness tingled my senses. The digital screen provided a display of all the options to prepare your coffee; extra dark, milk, cream, sugar, you name it, it was there. I decided to keep it simple, cappuccino with sweetener. The push on the screen activated a variety of mechanisms inside the big square metal box and a soft machinery sound started to radiate from it. Within minutes I was holding a freshly brewed cappuccino in my hand.

I brought the edge of the cup to my lips, my eyes closed, slowly sucking in the hot mixture, too hot to take a big swig, but cool enough to take small sips. The warmth combined with the scent of bitter sweetness of coffee, gave me a short-lived sense of comfort. My phone suddenly buzzed a short burst of vibrations. The table I had it placed on, seemed to function like a magnifier for the sound. It was a text message from a family member with an offer to stay the night with Becky here at the hospital, so I would be able to be with Connor and Dane at home. Since I wanted to give other people a break from taking care of the boys, I thought it would be a great plan.

"OK, see you tonight" I responded.

My mind wandered off to my possible activities for that night, for sure I would take the boys out for dinner somewhere.

I needed to refresh my cappuccino. I placed both my hands on the armrests of the chair to push myself up. After I climbed out of the chair, I turned around and grabbed my empty cup. The cappuccino machine was patiently waiting for me to select another beverage, when the door to the waiting room suddenly opened and a female voice announced,

"Mister Slootheer?!"

Shocked to hear my name, I put the paper coffee cup down on the counter and walked over to the lady in the blue scrubs that had just called my name. The clock right above the door caught my attention and I noticed it had only been 20 minutes since I left Becky in the MRI room.

"Already done?" I asked the nurse as I stepped closer to her.

She stepped aside from the door opening but kept her hand on the door to keep it open for me. When I passed through the opening, she let go and the door slowly closed behind us.

"No, we had to stop with the MRI, your wife is really upset," she explained as she walked in front of me.

Becky was waiting for me in her bed. She was curled up on her side, her hands close to her face, shivering. The moment she saw me walking towards her, she started to sit upright, stretching her arms out towards me.

"I couldn't do it babe," she immediately told me, while I was still walking towards her.

"I am so sorry," she continued.

Her eyes red from crying, still glittering in the light. She welcomed me into her arms, our lips kissed.

"Don't be sorry sweetie, you are fine," I said.

Her shoulders started to shrug, and more tears came down her face again, softly landing on my shoulder.

"It's ok honey, don't worry about it," I said.

I was trying to calm her down by rocking her gently back and forth. I kissed her on her cheek and tasted the sad saltiness from her tears. Her shoulders started to relax, no more tears of fear, anxiety, and frustration. She seemed to settle down.

The technician explained that he was able to complete most of the MRI of the neck, but that the last part of the brain 'failed' because they had to abort the procedure.

"I am not going back in there," Becky immediately burst out with a broken voice, pointing in the direction of the MRI room.

"I think we are done with the MRI," I said, "and we are ready to go back to our room now."

He understood that this was not a request. It was clear that Becky was not doing this again. He nodded, gave a gentle smile, and then he confirmed,

"Let me call transport for you guys."

Becky slowed down her breathing and calmness seemed to take over and settled her excitement. My hand glided over the sheet towards her, palm up, hand open. It connected with hers, the fear was still lingering in her eyes. It seemed that all her fear and despair was piling up and all came out at this moment right here. She found calmness in my arms, comfort knowing I would do anything in my power to protect her and help her fight this demon.

The Emergency Department was busy as usual. Medical staff was walking around, patients filled up all the rooms, some nurses were standing while others were sitting down at their workstations. Many recognized me the moment I walked into the ER. Some waved and smiled but kept walking, while others stopped what they were doing and came over to show their concern and care.

When you work in the ER, you go through a lot of emotional disasters that will leave an imprint on your soul for many years. A destructive motor vehicle crash, traumas with amputated limbs, or a dying child while your hands are on his chest in a rapid pace to keep his heart going. These are just a few of the many moments that will impact the rest of your life. As nurses, you rely on each other, you fall back onto the shoulders of the other nurse. When you lose it for a moment and break down in tears, they are there to offer a shoulder, a hug, or just an arm around you with a moment of silence.

A strong bond is created between all that work close in such a setting, and then when one of them is facing personal calamities, such as a sick spouse or child, the bond gets tighter and the urge to help grows. Many of the nurses came over to give a hug, no words were said, no words needed, their show of support explained it all. It is heartbreaking and heartwarming to see the compassion.

Tonight, I came down to the ER, to discuss Becky's MRI results with one of the ER docs. Earlier, when I was sitting in Becky's room while she was asleep, I noticed the floor nurse placing a report into Becky's chart. I was hoping it was the MRI report, and that it provided some answers about Becky's neck pain. It was placed under the tab 'imaging.'

My eyes were scanning the paper from left to right, reading the many terms used by medical professionals. I started to flip through the pages, searching for the heading of *'impression.'* There I would find the summary of all the aspects of the MRI, especially the abnormal ones.

I stood there motionless, my eyes rapidly moving, reading the sentences. Several words in the 'impression' section stood out and caused confusion: *'leptomeningeal metastasis.'* My brain searched for recognition of these words, nothing in my memory banks recalled what the diagnosis of leptomeningeal metastasis could mean; I had no clue.

I knew that *'metastasis'* is the spreading of cancer cells, but I did not know what *'leptomeningeal'* meant. Since Becky was still sound asleep, I decided to go downstairs to the ER to discuss this with one of the ER docs.

After the warm welcome from some of my fellow nurses, I walked over to the small office right behind the nurses' station where the ER doctors were sitting. I recognized the back of Doctor Carreon; short dark hair, tan skin, skinny posture. Silently I moved closer, I rested my hand on his shoulder, "Hey C, what's up?" I asked.

His left hand reached over to his right shoulder where my hand was. He placed his hand on top of mine and tapped it several times. Slowly he turned his head in my direction and smiled,

"How are you buddy?"

His chair rotated until he was facing me directly, resting his elbows on the armrests, his fingers folded together holding his hands interlocked. His eyes and silence proved he was waiting for an honest answer, he wanted to know how things were.

"Well, we're back. Becky had massive neck pains and they did an MRI earlier to see what is going on," I said.

"Any results yet?" he asked.

"Well, yes, leptomeningeal metastases, but I have no clue what that is. Do you?" I asked.

"Not sure about that," he said, "oncology is not my forte, but go check it out on 'up-to-date', they have the latest information."

After I sat down and logged in to the system, the screen provided links to research options. My right hand was holding on to the mouse. I made small, but deliberate movements, several clicks caused the 'up-to-date' website to open. My fingers tapped rapidly on the keyboard, making soft clicking noises. Letters appeared on the screen in the search-bar: 'Leptomeningeal Metastasis.' Within seconds, a list appeared with many research articles. I moved the small arrow on the screen over the first article heading, and with a simple click it opened up.

Again, my eyes were moving fast, from left to right and back, trying to detect the most important words that would give me a better understanding of what 'leptomeningeal' exactly could mean. As my eyes scanned the information, I was picking up key words. As I commenced gathering these words, my heart rate increased, the pounding sounds were louder with each beat in my ears, my stomach started to turn, all the words were doom and gloom, increasing negativity with every additional piece of information.

I didn't want these words, I was not prepared for this, Becky was not ready for this, this was not fair, this was not right. I wanted to close the article and walk away, but I had to know, reading the words; *median survival 4 to 6 weeks, incurable, rare form of metastasis, intrathecal chemotherapy, painful, death inevitable.*

Sharp knives were penetrating my soul, every word, another stab, deeper and deeper. The pain was unbearable, the blows imminent. A shiver inside took over as my brain absorbed the words of disaster. A lump formed in my throat and my stomach turned upside down. My whole world crumbled into nothing but rubble; everything fell out of place as the unexpected catastrophic words broke down my hope.

The silence from my lips and the blank stare at the computer screen must have warned Doctor Carreon about the doom that was overtaking my world, tearing out my soul. His gentle kind voice penetrated through my walls and pulled me back to reality.

"Everything ok?" he asked.

My response was slow, but clear.

"Not so sure C. Look at this research study," as I pointed my finger to the screen.

He stood up from his chair and came over. He placed his left hand on my right shoulder, leaned over to get closer at the screen, his face right next to mine. He took a rapid breath in and exhaled slowly. I knew he was preparing a response in his mind; he was trying to package this in a gentle way. Without deviating his eyes from the screen, his hand still on my shoulder, another long breath in, he started.

"Well, I am not an oncologist, so I am not sure, but," he paused, "this does not look good."

A soft squeeze from his hand on my shoulder confirmed his worry.

"I know," was all I could force to come out.

I walked back to Becky's room, my heart heavy, shoulders dropped down, eyes looking to the ground, breathing deep. Many people were in the hallways, but to me, sounds were gone, lights were dim, and it felt like I was walking alone by myself. No one else there, everything faded away and blurred out. My mind raced in circles trying to figure out if I should bring this news.

What if I am wrong? What if it is something else? What if there is a cure for it now?

I took the stairs, away from people, away from the world, I needed time to think, and walking up eight floors would do just that.

As I reached the oncology floor, I pushed the large heavy fire-door open. I still did not exactly understand what this new development meant. I decided not to say anything to Becky, I could not because I was not sure. Even though it felt wrong not to say anything, I could not take the risk to give her any wrong information. It had to come from Doctor Freeman; he knew what the consequences were from this discovery, and what available treatment was.

As I placed my hand on the door that would lead to Becky's room, I could hear her talking to someone. The door surface was cold, I pushed it inwards and stepped through the opening, into the room. The door opening was like a portal. In slow-motion my body glided through this gateway, and as I passed the metal posts, I waded through an invisible membrane, changing my appearance from quiet and worried to upbeat and elevated, as I usually was. For Becky's sake, I could not let her see my worries, I needed to stay strong for her. I could not allow her to think that I was doubting anything.

With a smile I plunged into her room, as chipper as always, I rectified my posture, straight up and joyful. I explained I went down to the ER just to chat with some of my colleagues.

"That's ok babe," Becky responded.

My outside was fake, happy, positive, and upbeat. My insides were screaming, pounding on the walls, mad, depressed, and down. My soul wept, the information from the MRI was destructive. I could barely keep myself standing up straight. I wanted to grab Becky in my arms, hold her tight, scream from the top of my lungs, and let my tears of pain flow down over her shoulder, telling her that I was sorry I let her down, tell her I didn't want her to die, to tell her I could not live without her ... but I couldn't. I had to stay strong. Strong for her, her steady rock in this tidal wave of disaster.

My kiss goodbye tonight felt different, I felt like Judas. It felt like I betrayed her by not telling her about the results. I know that not saying anything was the right thing to do - my uneducated knowledge of this development forced my silence, but emotionally, I wanted to tell her.

Our lips pressed together, my hand gentle on the side of her face, allowing our souls to flow together in an ocean of love, perfection, and understanding. Seconds felt like hours. No movement, no sounds, eyes closed, complete silence, perfect love.

"I love you, " I said after our lips detached.

Our commitment to each other was stronger than anyone would ever understand.

"I will be back early tomorrow morning to be here when Doctor Freeman comes in for his rounds," I promised her, not knowing the short night I was facing.

"Ok sweetie, I will be right here," she responded with a smile.

My body turned around and right before I disappeared through the door opening, I looked over my left shoulder towards her. Our eyes were like magnets, interlocked, my lips making a kissing sound.

"Love you sweetie," I added.

Her hand raised up towards her mouth, placed a soft loving kiss on the tips of her fingers, flattened out her hand and blew that perfectness towards me.

"Love you babe" she said.

I disappeared into the darkness of the hallway.

Thirteen

Fall was in full swing. Most trees had lost their beautiful colored leaves already, but some stragglers were still holding on, trying to ignore their inevitable detachment. The temperature during the day was getting closer to freezing, but at night it had already dipped below it a few times. Snow had not yet appeared, but it would not be much longer before that white flaky wetness would arrive. It was always welcomed by kids but cursed by those who have to drive in it or clean the sidewalks and driveways. It was always a fun sight to see Connor and Dane run out of the house, jumping around in that innocent white blanket, faces aimed at the sky, mouths wide open, catching snowflakes with their tongues. Becky would always collect the fresh snow and make little balls of it, then pour some liquid flavoring over them, creating homemade snow cones.

Tonight was a clear cold night and when I stepped outside, the chilling breeze shocked the skin on my face. It felt like pins and needles, my whole body shivered. With both hands I pulled up the collar of my jacket to cover my neck and ears. I started to walk faster to get to my truck as quickly as possible. From a distance I remote-started it to get the heater going. I was hoping for some temperature improvement by the time I arrived in the driver's seat. I realized that, when I sat down on the cold fabric of the seat, it hadn't really worked very well. The cold air was blasting from the dashboard up, ricocheting from the frozen windshield, into the cabin. It almost felt colder inside the truck than outside.

The headlights cut through the dark cold night, providing a path that guided me home. I was on autopilot from the moment I left the employee parking lot. For whatever reason, my brain was clearer and more open for thoughts when I was driving. My hands were on the wheel and my eyes stared into the dark night, mindless and numb, following wherever my headlights would shine.

A pressing urgency welled up inside me, I needed answers, I needed solutions, I needed knowledge. I knew that I would not sleep until I had satisfied my urge for information. The road was long and dark, but once I arrived back home, the welcoming committee was an absolute blessing. Both boys were in my arms, hugs and kisses created a joy in my heart that made me forget about the disaster from earlier. Lisa had already fed the boys, showered them, and they were in their pajamas ready for bed.

The TV was throwing colored pictures around the living room, the sound low to a soft mumble. The boys sat with me in the large chair, Dane on the left, Connor on the right. The painful question came from Dane this time.

"How is Mama doing, Papa?"

His words pierced through my skin into my already bleeding heart.

I can't tell them anything yet, I thought.

I explained that Mama was doing ok, but that they had to run some more tests to figure out why she had so much pain in her neck. I was still not sure about the impact of this leptomeningeal metastasis 'thing'.

As I was taking the boys to bed, Lisa decided to stay for a while so we could talk. Both boys were cuddled up in their beds, comforters pulled over their shoulders, close to their chin, ready to start snoozing like little puppies. As I walked by Lisa, I placed my hand on her shoulder and thanked her for her help that night.

"Oh, I just love to hang with the boys more than you realize," she responded.

I walked over to my chair, but before I could sit down, Lisa fired the loaded question,

"How is Beck doing?"

My body fell into the seat and I placed my legs on the ottoman, one at a time. Both my hands on my face, pulling down slowly as if I was trying to pull it off.

"Well," I said with a delicate crack in my voice, "things are not looking so good."

I retracted my feet from the ottoman, leaned forward, placed my elbows on my knees, and started to explain about the discovery I made earlier that evening from the MRI report.

Lisa was shocked and unsure how to react.

"Well, there might be a cure for it by now," she said hopefully.

I was hoping the same, but the research articles I read at the hospital were always new studies and in line with the latest developments. The four-to-six-week life expectancy continued to linger in my head, beating against my skull like a hammer with an intense unavoidable violence. I knew my mission for the night. I knew what I had to do before I would even think about sleep; I needed to research. I needed to know everything possible about this *leptomeningeal metastasis* issue.

"I will be back tomorrow morning at five thirty," Lisa promised, "so you can get there before Freeman does his morning rounds."

"Thank you, Lisa," I said.

The aroma of freshly made coffee had filled the kitchen. A single spoon laying on the counter with a torn package of sweetener laying right next to it. A trace of coffee created a small pool inside the bowl of the spoon, still releasing a minute amount of steam, confirming it was recently used for stirring. The light above the pine-colored wooden dining room table dropped bright illumination onto the surface where my laptop was waiting. The screen showed nothing but the logo from the manufacturer, slowly moving diagonally from side to side. Then, as it reached the edges of the screen, it bounced back to the other side. A subtle reflection could be seen on the glass from the sliding door that led to the deck at the back of the house.

I was sitting there, outside in the chilling darkness of the night. My fingers folded around my coffee mug, filled with warm freshly brewed caffeine. The steaming flavors floated into the cold air, providing my hands with needed warmth. My head relaxed back, my eyes gazing at the stars stuck in the darkness of the night. The cold air stroked my skin, and although it was refreshing, it was on the verge of being too cold, but I tolerated its frostiness with ease. I was preparing myself for the upcoming battle with my computer. I needed to find additional information and continue my search for possible solutions.

Slowly my mind drifted off to one of the first moments of our love. Becky and I had only been dating for a couple of months when she went on a trip with her family. A cruise down the Mississippi river from St. Louis to New Orleans on an old paddle-wheel steamboat. The day of her departure, she was leaving on an early morning flight.

Back in 1998, you could still walk up to the gateway as a non-passenger, this was 3 year before 9-11 happened. There was minimal security at the airport and there were not many restrictions for non-passengers, except that you could not get on the plane without a boarding pass.

The day Becky was leaving, I walked with her up to the gate. After she checked in, we kissed, said goodbye and off she went. I stood motionless while she slowly faded into the bridgeway leading to the airplane. After she disappeared around the corner, I waited for a brief moment, just to make sure she was gone.

With a big smile on my face I turned around and, as I started to peel my backpack off my shoulders, I walked up to the gate-agent that had just checked her in. She stared at me with big confusing eyes, her head slightly tilted to the right, eyebrows frowning,

"Can I help you sir?" she asked.

I explained to her that Becky was my girlfriend and that I had a small present for her. I pulled out a book, a card, some wrapping paper, and a single red rose from my backpack. I placed it all in front of her, on top of the counter. I continued my confession and informed her that I was hoping she would be willing to give this present to one of the flight attendants, so they could present my gift to my girl in seat 17A during the flight. Her frown changed to a big smile on her face, her eyes started to sparkle, her response exactly what I was hoping for.

"Aww ... that is so sweet! Of course, I will do that."

I placed the card on top of the book, then folded the wrapping paper around the book and card, placed the red rose on top of the package and handed it to her. She grabbed the wrapped gift with the rose and, with a glitter in her eyes almost revealing her emotions, she confirmed,

"I will take it to the flight attendant right now," as she vanished on the walkway to the plane.

Later that day my phone rang. It was Becky to inform me that she landed safely. Her voice was ecstatic.

"Oh my God!" she exclaimed.

"We are in the middle of the flight and this flight attendant comes up to me asking me if I was Miss Stagner?"

While Becky continued to elaborate about her experience mid-air, my heart jumped, and my soul roared. Exactly what I was hoping for, just happened.

The next surprise I had arranged was going to happen at the end of her steamboat trip. I purchased a plane ticket to New Orleans, rented a car, and arranged a hotel stay. Before Becky left, she gave me her travel itinerary. So, I knew where she was going and when she would be stopping at certain locations. There were many planned stops along the Mississippi River. The last stop, before arriving in New Orleans, was 'Houmas House and Gardens'. She would arrive there early afternoon on Friday. They would be stopping there for several hours so people were able to visit this historic place. It was there I had planned my next surprise.

After I flew into New Orleans early that morning, I picked up my rental car. Next stop would be a florist to obtain a bouquet of 24 red roses because 12 would just not be enough. With the roses comfortably positioned on the back seat of the rental sedan, I found my way to 'Houmas House', just about an hour drive following the Mississippi up north.

As I got closer, my heart was pounding. Excitement took over my senses. I was happy and nervous at the same time.

How would she react? Would she be mad? Happy? Surprised? Am I going too far? I shook my head, trying to shake it off to clear my thoughts.

I parked the rental in the almost empty parking lot. I leaned back and grabbed the roses before stepping out of the car. The gravel under the soles of my shoes made a grinding noise as I walked towards the 'Houmas House'. I realized that I had absolutely no idea where this boat would be stopping. It could be miles down or up the river and then maybe they would bus people here? My mind kept second-guessing my actions.

A lady that was purposefully positioned by the entrance, was going to be my source of information. As I walked up to her, she noticed me coming in her direction. She first looked me straight in the eyes, then slowly her eyes started to fall down towards my right arm. The red roses were secured between my forearm and body. As she noticed the flowers, she smiled. I smiled back at her and started to clarify my attendance.

"Good morning," I said.

She responded with a delicate nod, gentle smile, and a soft "Good morning."

"I am meeting my girlfriend here. She is on the paddle-wheel steamboat that will be stopping here this afternoon," I explained.

Her smile now bigger, she turned her body while she pointed just past the house.

"They will be docking over there," she explained.

Relieved that it was close by, I thanked the lady and started my walk towards the area where she had pointed. As I got closer, I noticed a path that crawled up the grass-covered dyke to the top of the levee. From there I saw an area on the side of the river that seemed suitable for a boat to dock. Patiently, I positioned myself at the highest point, standing motionless in beautiful green grass, flowers in my arms, gazing up the Mississippi river, waiting for her arrival.

Suddenly a large boat came floating from around the bend of the river, slowly moving through the water. My heart pounded faster, drumming in my ears. Excited and scared at the same time, a nervous smile uncontrollably appeared on my face. My eyes focused on the different deck layers to see if I could recognize anyone. Casually the large vessel passed by, floating towards the docking area.

People were standing on different decks, searching for where they would be docking. Hundreds of eyes were piercing down at me, the only person standing on a green grassy dyke, holding dark red flowers in my arms, as if he were holding a baby, with a nervous smile on his face.

The boat came to a halt and ropes were securely fastened around the large wooden beams sticking up from the water. As a metal walkway was pushed out from the second deck, I started to make my way down, slowly through the grass, towards the bridge that would bring me to my girl. Nervous about how she would react, but determined about my own feelings, I pushed forward. Suddenly a voice from one of the decks, somewhere onboard, became very clear.

"Who is that guy with those flowers?"

Not long after that question was launched, I placed my feet on the metal walkway. It was then when I heard her voice, excited, joyful, and surprised.

"Oh my God, oh my God! That's my man."

It was Becky, she recognized me. Her voice echoed over the calm Mississippi river waters, revealing her true affection. Her excitement to see me caused my nervousness to fade instantly. I arrived onboard and faced a large metal spiral staircase going up to all the different decks. While my brain tried to figure out which deck to go to, the solution arrived as I could hear footsteps, her footsteps, running on the metal steps, faster and faster, down the staircase.

I looked up and my heart swelled up so big that it wanted to explode from my chest. My smile was bigger than ever, my eyes sparkled tears of joy. There she was, running as fast as she could, down the metal stairs, circling down, faster and faster, her steps rapping loud on the metal stair. Her voice repeated,

"Oh my God...oh my God."

She arrived at the same floor where I was standing, but she was not slowing down. She continued at the same speed, coming towards me, flying towards me. She arrived in my arms, squeezed her body close to mine, her smell intoxicated my senses, her body was warm and soft.

"Hey babe," I said, "I have some flowers for you."

She looked up, her emerald green eyes shining beautiful, saying more than words could ever possibly say. All my fears and insecurities melted away with the gentle stroke of her hand along my face, right before her tender sweet lips touched mine.

Suddenly, a freezing cold breeze ripped me away from my memories and back to the present. My eyes slowly opened and the dark night pushed the realization of the current situation in front of me. The frigid winds increased, and as I stood up to find warmth inside the house, my shoulders automatically shrugged towards my neck, and a shiver ran along my spine. I reached out to ensure my coffee mug would travel with me. The sliding door opened with ease and a pleasant warmth surrounded me, welcoming my cold body back into the house. I stepped through the opening, turned around and closed the door softly, trying not to awake my boys.

Even though the warm air inside the house caressed my body, I continued to have shivers. I realized that I had been outside for too long. A soft red-and-black-blocked flannel shirt, a Christmas present from a couple of years ago, was hanging over the dining room chair.

I slipped one arm at a time inside the sleeves and folded the flannel shirt around my chest.

The screen stared at me with a curious silence. It wanted to help, it wanted me to search for answers. I placed my fingers on top of the keyboard and mindlessly I gazed at the screen. I was wondering what to search for. As I tilted my head to the side, it seemed to awaken logic. *'Leptomeningeal metastasis'* flew from my fingers onto the keyboard, placing those two words in the search bar. Many results appeared on the screen. Not much new information was revealed, still the same depressive outcome. No cure, four to six weeks life expectancy. I needed more information, more knowledge, and so the search began.

My eyes were scanning the words on the screen, running from left to right and back. Absorbing information like a dried-up sponge sucks up water after it had been laying in the sun too long. Research article after research article, studies, trails, opinions from oncologists, all resulted in the same final outcome: death within four to six weeks.

The only treatment to prolong this short time frame was intrathecal chemotherapy. With this type of treatment, chemotherapy would be infused directly into the spine, to soak the spinal cord and the spinal fluid in this poisonous solution. This treatment could prolong life for up to three months, but at the horrible price of barbaric pains. It was not recommended since there would be no quality of life.

My eyes gleamed to the left, noticing the time on my watch, 12:06, just past midnight. I had been on the research mission for a couple of hours now. I peeled my fingers off the keyboard and unglued my eyes from the screen. I leaned backwards, and as I closed my eyes, a slight burning sensation alarmed me that I had been staring at the screen too long. I placed both hands on my face and rubbed my fingers over my eyes several times, trying to wipe it off. I stretched my shoulders and stood up from the chair and walked over to the kitchen counter.

There was still some coffee in the pot. As I brought the pot closer to my nostrils, the stench elevated my senses to alarming levels. It was way past its due date. A quick dump into the sink followed by a clean water rinse eliminated the horrendous odor rapidly. A large glass of ice water was the next option for hydration. My lips welcomed the cool refreshing flow of water rolling down my throat and created a renewed feeling of energy. With my fingers placed back onto the keyboard, my eyes focused, I was ready for more research.

Results started to appear, but nothing new came to the surface. Again, all the studies resulted in the same depressing single option of spinal chemotherapy. Desperation fell over me, my face grim, my heart heavy. I read every article, every study, oncology websites, and research papers. None provided a solution; none provided a glimpse of hope. I folded my arms, let out a deep sigh, and stared at the screen with hollow eyes. My mind was numb and empty. No matter what I searched for, no matter what words I used, the results were all the same. The cursor blinked helplessly on my screen, my hands on my face gently rubbing my skin, trying to think, trying to proceed, trying to find a solution.

A sudden jolt straightened my back, as if someone injected me with new energy. My hands flew back onto the keyboard. A big gulp of cold water cleared my focus. I was no longer entering words in the search bar but started to dig deeper into the research articles. I knew that studies were frequently based on previous research, so I pulled up those older articles that were referenced in these newer studies.

Technology is amazing since it allowed me to access the older reports by a simple click on their title. I was clicking, reading, clicking, reading more. The flow of information was limitless. The reference links pulled me towards different articles from different medical professional journals.

It was 1:40 in the morning but I got this sudden burst of energy to keep me going. I was unable to stop. Suddenly a headline caught my attention - *'Effective treatment for some patients with leptomeningeal metastases.'* A simple click on the title brought me to another website where the posting was initially placed. Then, another link inside this posting pulled up the article that I had been looking for, the article that was placed onto my path for me to find.

Dr. Mark Socinski, a thoracic oncologist, published an article in the 'Journal of Clinical Oncology' in 2009, titled, *'Carcinomatous Meningitis in Non-Small-Cell lung cancer: Response to high-dose Erlotinib.'* In his research he described a case of a patient that was similar to Becky's situation. Socinski explained he was *'pulse-dosing'* Erlotinib (the generic name for Tarceva). Instead of giving the patient 150mg Tarceva once daily, he was administering 600mg once every four days. This caused an oversaturation of the cells with the medication, resulting in a higher blood-brain barrier penetration.

The schematics of this treatment plan will become complex for those without medical training, so let me explain:

Around the spinal cord and brain is a protective barrier that is called the 'blood-brain-barrier.' The purpose of this barrier is to keep 'bad' elements out of the brain, spinal cord, and spinal fluid. Most medications will not pass this barrier, but Tarceva (Erlotinib) has some penetration and as such it would actually penetrate the brain, spinal cord, and spinal fluid.

When a person has leptomeningeal metastasis, the cancer cells are active inside of this blood-brain barrier. So, by oversaturating the cells on the outside of the spinal cord, there is a higher potential for penetration through this protective layer. Socinski's goal was to have more Tarceva passing through the barrier, and with a 600mg dose once every four days he tried to accomplish just that. The patient in his study surpassed the life expectancy of four to six weeks. She stayed on this high dose of Tarceva for a total of ten months and lived for a total of 24 months, compared to six weeks.

My heart pounded from excitement. An enormous surge of vigor pulsated through my body.

'I FOUND IT!' I yelled in my mind while making a balled raised fist as a sign of victory.

I knew this would not cure Becky, but I knew it would provide for more time. More time would allow more healing. Maybe more time for new research or medical developments. I planned to bring up this research to Doctor Freeman during his morning rounds the following day.

Parking at the hospital was easy in the early morning hours. Shift-change would not happen for another hour, so only the night shift people would be here at this time. I decided not to take the employee entrance because I did not feel like talking to anyone that morning. As I got closer to the sliding doors, both slid open with a soft swooshing sound. This early in the morning, the main entrance was still closed and everyone had to come in through the ER entrance.

The ER waiting room was almost empty, just two people were curled up on seats with a pillow and blanket. Frequently, family members of ER patients would find refuge here in the waiting room. Just to get a quick nap since they had been awake all night.

The triage nurse was not at her station, but the receptionist recognized me. She smiled and raised her hand, waving at me. I returned the smile and gave a quick elevation of my hand, but continued my walk. I wanted to get to Becky's room as fast as possible, so I avoided any conversation with her.

The long hallway towards the elevators led past the stalls for admission. It was normally filled with people, but at this hour it was completely empty and abandoned. The silence of this usually busy place gave an eerie feeling, almost like walking through a ghost town.

All three of the elevator doors were open. This could have been a great scene for a horror movie where, if you entered the wrong elevator, you would plummet to the burning fires of hell. Regardless of the possible 'plummeting to hell' thought, I stepped into the first one. Within seconds a large metal door slid out from its hiding place inside the wall and entrapped me inside. The soft 'ping' sound confirmed that the door was closed. It seemed comical given the nature of the scary movie approach; a soft gentle ping followed by the flames of hell nibbling at your legs.

A tap on the rounded push-button with a large '8' on it, caused it to light up with a soft glow and started the elevator into an upward motion. A sudden rapid deceleration brought the elevator to a hasty halt on the eighth floor and it spit me out onto the freshly cleaned and shiny linoleum. The strong odor of fresh pine mixed with some kind of chemical cleaner burned the inside of my nostrils, indicating that the floor was cleaned and polished recently.

Before I turned into the hallway of the oncology floor, the sound of many voices traveled rapidly towards me. Many nurses were hovering around the nurses' station. They were probably excited that their nightshift was almost over, and they could crawl into their warm beds for some well-deserved sleep.

The physicians had started their morning rounds and, as usual, new orders for labs, x-rays, treatments, and medicine would keep the nurses busy for just a little longer before they could clock out. As I made my way there, their voices became louder.

A large clock behind the counter where the floor charge-nurse was sitting displayed the digital time: 06:11AM. I slowed down, and as I came to a halt at the station, I placed both of my hands on top of the counter as if I were going to order food. The charge nurse looked at me, maintained her optimism even though she was tired, and smiled. With a friendly and crisp voice, she acknowledged my arrival.

"Good morning Roy."

I smiled back while thinking that it was sad that you are known by name by the nurses on the oncology floor because you have been there so many times.

"Has Doctor Freeman arrived yet?" I asked.

"He got here a couple of minutes ago," she responded, "but I don't think he went to see Becky yet."

"Great, thank you."

I proceeded with my journey to Becky's room.

The hallway was busy. Fast moving shoes hit the ground like a military parade. The many nurses, doctors, and their assistants crowded the long corridor with doors left and right that would lead to each individual patient room. Many voices conversed in different tones and sounds, creating a buzzing chatter like you would hear at birthday parties and overcrowded bars. I was dodging people while I tried to make my way to Becky's room. My shoes made high- pitched squeaking noises as I had to make unexpected turns and twists. As my eyes peeled through the crowds, I saw Doctor Freeman standing at the desk by Becky's room. Angie, his nurse, was standing next to him. She was talking to him while he was flipping through the pages of Becky's medical file.

"Good Morning," I exclaimed, trying to get their attention.

Both Doctor Freeman and Angie turned their heads, almost simultaneously as if they practiced it before.

"Good morning," they both responded.

Doctor Freeman's face did not release a smile. His eyes were almost stern. Normally he was always positive and chipper, but today he was quiet and seemed concerned.

Angie, as usual, was pleasant and positive. She was amazing at her job, always trying to cheer you up no matter how bad the situation was.

I looked Doctor Freeman straight in the eyes, my body motionless.

"Is it what I think it is? Is it this bad?" I asked him.

The blank stare on his face, his eyes not expressing anything, the silence was painstaking.

"Let's go inside," he said, as he made a waving gesture with his hand, open palm, towards the door, inviting me to go inside Becky's room.

Fourteen

Becky was sitting straight up in bed. My heart was thumping in my chest so hard I could feel the pulse in my carotid arteries. This was the moment of truth, now the news would be brought to Becky. Although the secret was trapped inside me for only a short time, it was still too long.

When I walked through the door, Becky's eyes lit up, a big smile came on her face, and she opened up her arms for a hug.

"Hey babe," she said.

Her amazingly positive attitude, topped with those big green eyes, was irresistible. I walked over to the bed, leaned forward and right before we sealed our love with a kiss, I replied,

"Morning sweetie."

"And look who is here," she joyfully announced when she noticed that Doctor Freeman walked in right behind me.

He placed himself at the end of the bed, both hands with fingers interlocked in front of him. Angie was right next to him but a little further to the back, smiling and waving at Becky.

"Morning," she whispered.

Becky responded with a wave back.

"Good morning Becky, how are you feeling today?" Doctor Freeman asked.

"I had a pretty good night," Becky said, "this pain-pump really helped a lot".

"Well the results of the MRI came in…"

As he paused, I took that opportunity to sit down next to Becky. I grabbed her left hand and held it in mine. Doctor Freeman's eyes became worrisome, his pupils tightened for controlled focus.

"Your neck pain is caused by the spreading from the cancer into your neck," he continued, "this is also known as leptomeningeal metastases."

Freeman shifted his posture to one leg, both his hands started to make gestures to support his words. Angie's stood motionless behind him. Her eyes spoke strong words of sympathy.

"This is a very rare development and the prognosis is not good."

I could feel my heart sinking deeper and deeper, a lump in my throat prevented any vocal responses, my stomach was in a knot. My hand felt a delicate squeeze from Becky's hand. Her eyes focused on Doctor Freeman, her body motionless.

"Since this is such a rare development, only 5% of lung-cancer patients get this, not much research has been done," he explained. "Ultimately, we are looking at four to six weeks. You might have till Christmas."

A silence so deafening and painful took over the room. Becky and I were staring at Doctor Freeman, his face motionless and grim. A miniscule glittering in the corner of his eye revealed that his emotions were welling up. He was no longer just an oncologist that was taking care of a patient, but a human being with feelings showing empathy and sadness. This was one of the reasons that Becky and I had chosen him as her oncologist. He truly cared.

Angie, still standing behind him, removed a tear from her eyes with her right index finger. Becky's hand was now squeezing mine tighter, her body remained motionless, her eyes still focused at him. Even though this moment only lasted seconds, it felt like hours. Becky continued to stay motionless, not a word was spoken.

Her head slowly turned towards me, her eyes screaming for help, her soul shivering inside. The desperate cry from her eyes was loud and filled with horror. My focus was on Becky, all other sounds faded as my focus intensified. Everything around her slowly evaporated. Her soul was clinging to mine. All I could see was her, no sounds, no vision.

Doctor Freeman broke the silence and disrupted the initial shock, cutting through the thick heavy atmosphere.

"Besides this development, they also found several tumors in your brain."

The onslaught continued. It was obvious this cancer was on a horrific path of destruction. Ruthless, it advanced to become victorious in its ultimate quest.

"They also noticed increased activity of the primary tumor in the left lung. It is increasing in size," Freeman explained.

"There is now also activity seen in the right lung," he continued.

It felt as if someone were beating us up with a baseball bat and would not stop.

After he described the magnitude of challenges ahead, since the cancer had spread to so many areas of her body, he explained that there were not many options. Radiation could control some of the growth in the lungs and neck, and of course we would continue with the Tarceva.

The only possible known treatment for the leptomeningeal metastases was intrathecal chemotherapy. Since this treatment was so painful, it would ravage any quality of life. Doctor Freeman recommended not to proceed with this option. The brain tumors could also be radiated with the precision 'cyber knife' treatment.

His muteness after he delivered the horrific news was painful. I knew that he had not expected this to happen.

"I will be back after my rounds," he said.

"That will give you both some time to think and talk about it."

He left the room quietly. Angie followed him silently. She looked at us, and although she did not say anything, the expression on her face spoke powerful words.

The door fell shut behind them. Silence filled the room. We just sat there, completely numb from the beating. Becky looked at me and the sadness in her eyes tore my soul apart. She was devastated. I could see and feel it. She looked at me for guidance. Her hand in mine, white knuckled, strong but scared. From the moment she was diagnosed, she had placed her trust in me, but we always decided together.

Her beautiful green eyes, as radiant as always, now covered with tears ripped through my soul like a hot knife through butter. She was waiting for me to come up with a solution.

"Sweetheart," I said, "last night I read the MRI report and I was aware of this situation." I took a deep breath in and continued.

"But I was not sure what it all meant. I even went downstairs to talk to one of the ER docs to explain the MRI, but he was not sure either."

Becky's eyes were soft, her attention glued to every word I spoke. Her body frozen, her voice silent.

"So, last night I researched almost everything that there is to know about leptomeningeal metastases," I explained, "and I found this very interesting research study that was completed several years ago that might give us some time and hope."

I tried to give her all the information I had. It was important for her to understand that the ultimate accomplishment of this treatment plan was time. After she soaked up all the information, she smiled and her eyes sparkled.

It must have been at least one hour before Doctor Freeman returned to the room. This time he was alone. Angie had already gone to the clinic to start the day there. His silence exposed his concern for this horrifying progress. Before he could say anything, I told him that I reviewed the MRI last night and that I was aware of the leptomeningeal metastasis.

"I spent many hours researching leptomeningeal metastases last night," I said, "and besides learning more about it than I ever wanted to know, I found a possible treatment that might give us more time."

His eyes confused, he tilted his head slightly to the left, and a delicate frown appeared. He continued to be silent, ready to hear what I'd discovered.

This was one of the characteristics I did really appreciate from him; his willingness to listen and to be open for discussion. Many other physicians would have pushed any input from a patient to the side. After all, they were the ones who went to medical school, they were the ones that studied for many years, and they were the ones who worked in this field. Arrogance is a character trait of some of these providers, but not with Doctor Freeman, he was always open for discussion and new ideas.

His silence confirmed that he was patiently waiting for me to present him with the information. My hand disappeared into the inside pocket of my black leather coat that was hanging over the wooden chair to my left. I pulled out a stack of papers. It was the research article.

"Here," I said as I handed the papers to him, "this is the study from Doctor Socinski."

His eyes flew rapidly over the words, flipping the pages over, his pupils moving quickly from left to right and back. When he was done reading it, he asked if he could keep the article.

"Of course," I replied.

"I will research this treatment plan in more detail," he said, "but as far as I can see now, I think we should go ahead and try it. There is not much else we can do."

Doctor Freeman explained that he met with Doctor Socinski several times when he was getting his degree from the University of Iowa. He told us that Socinski became one of the leading thoracic oncologists because of his out-of-the-box thinking and progressive treatment approaches.

In collaboration with Doctor Freeman, Becky and I decided that she would start the pulse-dosing of 600mg Tarceva once every four days gradually. First, she would start taking 300mg Tarceva every other day. Then, after a week, she would increase it to 450mg every third day. Finally, if all went well, she would start taking the 600mg, once every four days. It made Becky feel better to slowly move into the new plan.

Radiation would also become a part of the overall treatment approach. She would receive radiation of her neck to control the growth of the leptomeningeal metastasis, radiating of the chest to control the expansion of the initial tumor in Becky's left lung, and radiation of her head to control the brain cancer. This would help to shrink the tumors and slow down further growth.

The air was crisp and clear, the sun high in the sky. A gentle breeze with temperatures in the low 30s made it a perfect late fall afternoon. I turned onto the long driveway that led to Becky's mother's house. Each side of the concrete pathway was covered by tall trees, perfectly spaced in a single row. Although most of them were leafless at the moment, just a few short months ago they displayed beautiful colors of dark red, amber, and all tints of brown.

Many cars were parked in front of the double-door garage and the circle-drive at the front entrance of the house. Since I had called for the family meeting, I knew that they would all be here. I decided it was important to relay all the information to the family members personally. It was important for them to be informed of the latest developments and the altered treatment plan.

My fingers folded around the bronze metal door-grip and pushed the large wooden door open. A gentle chime sounded as I stepped into the house. Straight ahead of me was the large dining room with a circular table in the middle, occupied by all family members waiting for me to arrive. It was an awkward situation and the tension was suffocating. You could feel it with every movement, every step, sticking on you like a hot humid summer day. We all knew this meeting was going to be painful, the one that no one wanted but it had to happen since there was no escaping from it. I sat down in the last empty chair that surrounded the table. Stillness was prevalent. All their eyes were aimed at me. I could feel their piercing looks for answers, maybe even guidance. It was one of the few times I actually had the feeling that they appreciated me for who I was, and for what I did.

I was staring at the table, my hands folded in front of me as if I was praying to God for strength and guidance. Seconds felt like minutes, minutes like hours. With a deep breath in my chest expanded to its maximum, followed by a full exhale. I lifted my eyes up from the table, giving everyone a fair amount of pupilar interaction.

"The results from the MRI yesterday are not good," I said.

Their eyes glued onto me, hanging on my words. They were all sitting paralyzed at the table, waiting for the information. As I started to explain the impact of the metastases into her neck and spinal cord, the movement from the cancer cells to her brain, right lung and worsening of the primary tumor, I noticed an increasing vibration in my voice. Deep inside me I wished I was just ignorant like everyone else. Not knowing all this medical stuff. I just wanted to be Becky's husband that would hold her hand and not worry about treatment plans, research, death, family members, or friends. Sometimes it is a blessing to be insignificant. As these thoughts punctured my brain, I broke down.

"I am failing her," I said. "I have tried so hard."

As I broke down, tears streamed from my eyes. I did not know how they saw me, but I knew that they were now aware that I was just human, with feelings, concerns, and needs.

The radiation nurse placed her hands on the handles of Becky's wheelchair. She leaned over, and while she looked at Becky, she clarified,

"I know where I am going, so allow me to get you there."

Her soft and friendly voice was combined with an addictive smile and allowed for no other option than to smile back at her and agree. As we maneuvered through a labyrinth of hallways, I noticed that they tried to give this area a 'homey-feeling.' The carpet was dark burgundy red, several side tables sat along the walls, and various pieces of art were creatively and purposefully placed throughout the treatment center. We finally came to a humongous door-opening, way too large for even an oversized door, and as we passed the door posts, my eyes caught the size of them. They were about two feet wide. It almost felt as if we walked into a safe at a bank. The nurse explained that these were specially designed doors lined with lead to keep the radiation inside the treatment room.

We were at the 'CyberKnife' facility to get measured for a mask that was going to be placed over Becky's face every time she came in for a radiation treatment of her brain. The mask helps to diminish the risk of movement during radiation and ensured the same placement of the head in relation to the radiation device. Accuracy is essential to eliminate the risk of radiating healthy tissue and making sure that exactly the same area gets 'hit' every time.

The mask was made of a plastic-gauze type material. They first heated it to make it soft and pliable. It was then stretched over Becky's face and attached to the table with some kind of plastic clips. The material took the shape of the contours of Becky's face and slowly hardened.

During the first treatment day, they also placed tattoo markings on Becky's chest. These were reference points for the radiation specialist to line up the machines before they started to radiate the tumors in her chest. Marking these locations with tattoos was the only option to ensure that they would not fade over time.

Inside the treatment room we were greeted by another radiation technician. As both technicians started to go through all the steps to get the mask fitted, they explained that every time Becky came in for treatment, the set-up would take up most of the time.

As they finished up their preparations, Becky was lying motionless on that cold, hard table with her face still attached to it. The tech explained to Becky that everyone would leave the room now, so they could start with the radiation. The technician waved at me, making the gesture to leave the room. Instead, I walked over to Becky and placed my hand in hers. She grabbed it with a strong grip and squeezed it tight. I knew she was scared, afraid of this procedure. Her face was covered with some plastic device, attached to the table, her eyes closed, and unable to move. I just stood there, staring at her, holding her hand.

"I love you babe," I said.

"Mhmhm," was all she could bring out since the mask made it impossible for her to talk.

"I will be right here, outside the room, okay?" I tried to reassure her that I was close by.

"Mhmhm," as she gave my hand a delicate squeeze.

I lowered my face and placed a single kiss on the back of her hand.

The moment I stepped out through that oversized door, it started to close behind me. When it fell into place, a large loud clicking noise confirmed the door was locked. The technician waved at me to come with him into the control room.

"You can come with us to the control room," the male technician said.

The lights were dim, a large row of computer screens was lined up against the wall. The screens displayed, in black and white, Becky's brain and her chest. In front of these screens were many buttons, knobs, sliding levers, and flashing lights. He pushed several buttons and explained,

"The machine is now lining up and will start radiation soon."

Becky was discharged on Friday afternoon. It was getting increasingly colder by the day. Winter had arrived with chilling temperatures below zero, painful wind chills, and plenty of snow. Today was a cloudy and miserably cold day. While the nurse was helping Becky get ready, I left to go ahead and pull the truck around to the main entrance.

Despite the fact that I had turned the heater in the truck to high, it was still blowing cold air in our faces when we left the hospital to go home. The engine was not warm enough yet, but soon it would provide us with a comfortable warm blast. Becky reached over the middle console with her left arm, grabbed my hand, and folded her fingers between mine. I quickly peeked her way, and as our eyes interlocked, I puckered my lips and blew her a kiss. Her beautiful smile arrived on her face and her eyes sparkled.

"I love you," she said, followed by a kiss to my hand.

We exchanged ideas and discussed the new treatment plan. I knew she was concerned about this, since she had some skin issues and massive episodes of diarrhea alternating with constipation caused by the side effects of Tarceva. I am sure she was scared that these side effects would quadruple if she increased the amount of medicine. Logical thinking would assume so, but it was for sure worth a try if it would prolong her life past the prognosis of four-to-six weeks.

"If the side-effects get too bad, we can always lower it again," I reassured her.

Becky agreed.

The house was wrapped in silence when we arrived. It was early afternoon so both Connor and Dane were still at school. My arm supported Becky as I guided her up the short set of steps. From there, the path became too narrow, with the TV on the right and couch on the left, to walk beside each other. I shifted my body in front of her, never letting go, but now I was walking backwards holding both her hands. She shuffled along the hardwood floor.

As she looked straight at me, the connection between our souls engaged to a higher level. Whenever our pupils linked, regardless of the misery she was in, regardless of the fear, the pain, and the insecurity about what was going to happen, she continued to have that amazing ability to look at me and make my heart beat faster. She never said anything, but that look, as brief as it could be, told me more than a thousand words.

We just looked and shuffled, me moving backwards, her moving forward, until we arrived at the chair. She came closer, her hand slowly raised up towards my face, a delicate touch released a chain reaction of peace and comfort inside me. Her face got close to mine, never losing eye contact until that moment right before our lips touched. As our eyes closed, it created a darkness filled with inner harmony and warm comfort of love. These moments with Becky were past the confusion of language. It was pure and clear inner communication of two souls that were meant to be together. Two souls so connected that there were no questions... ever.

She folded up her legs underneath her, grabbed the blanket that was hanging on the back of the seat, and wrapped it around her legs. She tapped her hand on the leather cushion next to her, inviting me to come over and sit.

"Let me make you some tea first, sweetie," I said.

Her big smile confirmed approval of my suggestion.

A sudden vibration of my phone in my jeans pocket alerted me of an incoming call.

"Hang on," I said, as I grabbed the phone and looked at the screen for the caller ID.

Since it had a different area code, I knew it was from out of state. Reluctantly I answered the call.

"Hello?"

A dark male voice on the other side responded,

"Hi there, is this Roy Sloot...Slother?" As usual, no one pronounced my name correctly the first time.

"Yes, it is," I answered. "Who is this?"

"This is Doctor Mark Socinski," he said.

"You called a couple of days ago and left a message with my nurse. I am returning your call."

My eyes sprang wide-open. I looked at Becky, and while holding the phone to my ear, I started to point at the phone with my index finger, and tried to speak without sound hoping she would be able to read my lips.

"IT IS DOCTOR SOCINSKI," I slowly spoke.

Becky, realizing that I was clearly super excited about something, raised her shoulders, both hands with palms in the air, looking at me confused. She did not understand my soundless language, and she was not able to read my lips. I placed my hand over the speaker of the phone, leaned forward closer to her, and whispered,

"It is Doctor Socinski, from the research article."

"Oh my God, he is calling you?" Becky softly said.

All I could do was nod and smile.

I informed him about Becky's diagnosis of stage IV cancer with the new development of leptomeningeal metastasis. I explained that I wanted to discuss the study he completed about pulse-dosing with Tarceva. He clarified that he was unable to give any treatment advice, since Becky was not his patient. I voiced my understanding of that dilemma but clarified that I also discussed this research article with Doctor Freeman, and that he was very intrigued by this treatment plan.

Doctor Socinski and I talked in great detail about the patient from the study that was published in 2009. We continued to discuss the effects of pulse-dosing and the details about the penetration of the blood brain barrier, and possible side-effects. I was so thankful for his return phone call. I never expected that anyone would call me back, let alone himself.

After about 30 minutes, we finished our conversation. I put my phone back in my pocket and looked at Becky full of excitement.

"Wow honey," I exclaimed, "that was awesome. That was Doctor Socinski!"

"Why did he call you babe?" Becky asked, still confused about why he reached out to me.

"Well," I said, "the other day, after we discussed this option for treatment, I just decided to call him."

Becky had this 'awe' look in her eyes, that I actually had the guts to pick up the phone and just call a person like that.

"I know, I know," I said, "no one else would do that, but I just did. I wanted to know if he had done any further research that might have been important to know. Sometimes it is just easier to talk to a person directly, instead of trying to research that on the web," I said, as I raised my shoulders like it was the most common thing to do.

Fifteen

Our home was filled with women; firefighter wives. All dressed in purple, talking over each other, laughing loudly, hugging, and crying. At times it sounded like a hen house, followed by the silence of falling tears. Only those who have military, law-enforcement, or firefighter families understand the comradery amongst those serving, and those who are married into that service. Most of my best friends were from the firehouse. Most of Becky's best friends were the spouses of those firefighters. It is a tight community with intense love and care for one another.

Several months ago, some of these firefighter wives decided to organize a fundraiser for Becky's benefit. It was their way of saying *'we care.'* Although they already showed us every day that they cared by being there for us when we needed anything, they wanted to do this.

Initially, when they brought up the plan for the fundraiser, Becky did not go for it. She didn't like to be the center of attention. She wanted to stay out of the spotlight, stay behind the scenes, and do things anonymously. But when she realized it was their way of saying *'we care and we want to do something'* she agreed to it. The name *'Becky's Crusaders - One for All, All for One'* was created. Everything was in purple, since it was Becky's favorite color. The day of the event was set to be on December 15th.

Becky was very much aware of the fact that everyone was expecting her to say something during the evening of the event, but she was terrified of public speaking. She would break out in cold sweats and have heart palpitations just by thinking about it. She looked at me one afternoon while she was lying in bed, holding on to my hand.

"Honey," she said, "you know I cannot do this."

"I know babe," I said while smiling.

She shook my hand to ensure I understood the seriousness of the situation.

"No, really babe, I can't," with a desperate tone in her voice.

My smile slowly faded, my face more serious, and with a normal voice I clarified my understanding.

"Babe, don't worry about it. I will stand up there and do your speech, but you have to write it, okay?"

A deal was made, and she was content with that solution.

At that time, Becky went through some rough spots as a result of all the brain radiation. It caused swelling of the brain, which caused her to suffer from severe headaches. To control them, they prescribed her large doses of prednisone for a prolonged period of time. This medication is a cortico-steroid that helped with the swelling, but one of the side effects is something known as 'moon-face' – because it caused swelling of the face, making it appear rounder.

Although Becky never said anything about it, I knew she was very upset with this 'moon-face' appearance. The other side-effect of steroids, like hunger, did not affect her. On the contrary, she continued to lose weight, and maybe her skinny body made that 'moon-face' look more prominent. We never spoke about it, we never mentioned it, but we both knew how she felt about it.

On the day of the event, she was nervous, but hid it very well. We were supposed to be there around 3:30 in the afternoon since the fund-raiser started at 4pm. It would last until eight that evening. We arrived on time at the local golf-course where the fundraiser was held. The owners were so kind to donate the building for us to use.

All the firefighters were there and it was good to see them all working together with their spouses to make this happening a success. Becky found a good spot to sit, close to the door, just in case she wanted to sneak out if she got tired and wanted to go home. Many people arrived between four and five. They all, of course, wanted to spend some time with Becky. When I saw her battery was draining pretty fast, I sat down next to her, placed my hand on her thigh, and leaned over to whisper in her ear.

"Are you doing ok babe?"

She turned her face towards me and touched my cheek with her hand.

"Just a little longer," she said.

Her eyes looked tired, her face was still all smiles, but I could see she was getting to the end of her rope.

"I will give the speech now, ok?"

She smiled, nodded, and sealed our agreement with a kiss.

As I stood up, I looked for one of the firefighter wives that was part of organizing this wonderful event. I scanned the area and found one; she was talking to another person but facing me. As soon as she noticed I was trying to connect with her, she came over.

"What's up?" she asked.

"I think I will do Becky's speech now," I told her, "and then we might go home pretty soon after that. Becky is getting tired."

"Okay," she responded, and took off to get me the microphone.

Within minutes she returned, the microphone in her hand as she stood right next to me. She gazed down at the handle of the microphone and, with her right thumb, moved the little switch in the middle from the 'off' to the 'on' position. She brought the microphone up and tapped on the screen. A loud banging sound was noted over the speakers. Instantly everyone stopped talking. Immediately I got the microphone stuffed in my hand, followed by a soft,

"Here you go," as she disappeared into the crowds

I smiled, folded my fingers around the handle, and realized that she too might have a fear of public speaking. I brought the microphone close to my mouth and started.

"Thank you all for being here tonight. Becky and I are very pleased to see so many people here and feel truly blessed with wonderful friends."

My eyes were glazing over the many people in the building, trying to make eye contact with everyone there. After I gave thanks for those who organized the event, I went into Becky's speech.

"Roy and I want to thank all of you who are here supporting us. You are our family and friends; you are our angels. When Roy and I started the journey of our lives together, we chose Altoona to be our home. We initially wanted to live here to be closer to our family. We found out quickly how a community of wonderful people can become family too.

The first group of people to win our hearts were the firefighters from the Altoona Fire Department. Shortly after settling in our new home, we had a scary medical emergency with Connor, who was still a newborn then. We called 911 and in the fastest response time ever (three minutes,) Larry Lawson had jumped the fence between our homes and was taking care of our Connor. Within five minutes more help arrived. Roy and I were so grateful, that the next day Roy felt so compelled to go and talk to the firefighters to thank them personally, and to become one of them. He wanted to be part of this amazing group of heroes ... and who doesn't like chili?

The day Roy joined the fire department, our family circle grew. It didn't just include the men and women that volunteered with him, it included their spouses, children, friends, and families. Our whole world got bigger and better because we met you.

Years passed and our family added another adventure to our journey, the Coffee House Hollander. Owning a business in Altoona gave us the opportunity to meet and interact with even more people in our community. The group of people that we met through the Chamber of Commerce became more than local business owners; they soon became part of our circle of friends.

Altoona is always growing, but to us it will always be a small town with a big heart. Every time one of the boys moved up a grade or joined a ball team, our lives became richer for having met each of you. The schools, the Shriners, banks, grocery stores, golf courses, restaurants, and the library...these aren't just buildings to us. These are places that have changed our lives because here in Altoona, we have found community. Community became friends and friends became family.

It is said that 'Altoona' is a native American word meaning 'high ground.' That may be true, but for Roy and me, Altoona will always mean 'a place where angels live.'

Thank you for being our angels. We love you."

I leaned over to my side and placed my hand on Becky's cheek. She looked at me with eyes filled with love. We kissed and she whispered,

"Let's go home babe, I am really tired."

I told one of the organizers that we were leaving and that we were going to sneak out the door. She walked with us to help Becky into the car. Not many noticed that we left, but that was part of the plan, otherwise it would have taken hours to leave. My phone pinged almost the whole way back home, many people were texting to say 'goodbye' and 'I love you guys.' It was amazing to have so many great, loving friends.

***

The fresh snow from the night before stuck to the world and gave everything a beautiful white and pure look. The ice-cold blistering wind caused a painful experience to any exposed skin, like frigid knives flying through the air. Any uncovered part of your body would cause you to immediately regret the decision to step outside. I snowplowed a path from the front door to my truck to minimize the risk of slipping and falling. Today we would go back to see Doctor Freeman to discuss the results of the latest MRI. It had been over two months since we started the pulse-dosing of Tarceva, and Doctor Freeman wanted to see how Becky was doing on this new plan.

It was amazing to realize that the side-effects she initially experienced with Tarceva, the skin problems and diarrhea, almost completely disappeared. We stayed in contact with Doctor Freeman and his nurse Angie weekly, just to give them updates or ask any questions we had.

Personally, I was stoked to see that the treatment plan of pulse-dosing with Tarceva was working. Two months ago, Doctor Freeman stood at Becky's bed in room 825 on 8-south making the devastating statement that she might make it to Christmas that year, only 6 weeks. That holiday was a month ago, so to me, this was a time for careful optimism, and we were excited to meet with Doctor Freeman to see what the latest MRI had to tell us.

Becky was sitting on our chair, all bundled up in a warm winter coat, scarf around her neck, warm knitted wool cap on her head. She started to lose her hair about a week ago. They told us at CyberKnife that the radiation of her brain would eventually cause hair loss. The radioactive rays would temporarily destroy the hair follicles, leading to baldness.

After all the radiation treatments were done, Becky's hair did not show any signs of thinning at all. I kept saying that Becky was the exception to the rule and that she would be spared from this depressive reminder of cancer. Last week though, we found big piles of hair on Becky's pillow. Whenever I would give her a bath, more hair would clog up the drain. It was a painful sight over which not many words were spilled. We kept it quiet, but we both knew that eventually all her hair would be gone. Right now, there were many bald spots and Becky already said,

"I am gonna get the clippers to it soon."

Her hair used to be thick and wavy, strong and fast-growing. The brutal radioactive attack was ruthless and without exception, yet another harsh experience of the relentless effect of the cancerous destruction of healthy human cells. It is the insecurity of what is going to happen next that eats you. Little victories followed by brutal fall backs. Little by little the cancer was sneaking through every cell in her body. It was taking over, giving a little bit back, then taking more. Hope is the only glue that tries to keep things together; hope for a cure, hope for a miracle, hope for more time.

I walked up the stairs to our living room after I started my truck, trying to pre-warm it for her. Becky despised the cold, she hated it with every cell of her body. Yet we lived in a state with very strong, cold winters. We always talked about moving to Florida, but until that actually happened, we went on vacation to the Florida Keys several times a year. We soaked up the sun, immersed ourselves in the salty ocean water, and recharged until we came back again.

Today was just another brutally cold day in Iowa. All bundled up myself, I placed my arm around her, helped her up from the chair, and we slowly walked over to the front door where we were greeted by the blistering cold.

"Oh my God!" were the only words Becky could blast out.

She curled up to me, using me as a shield to keep the frigid wind off of her; an assignment I proudly accepted. My arm strong around her, my body protecting her. We walked around the truck, I quickly opened her door, then guided her into the already warmed cabin. I closed her door rapidly to keep the cold blistering wind from hitting her body.

Fast paced I walked around to sit down in the driver's seat. Becky was sitting with both her hands close to her face, blowing warm air from her lungs onto them and rubbing them together for friction to cause more warmth.

"Oh my God honey, it is so cold," she said.

I looked over and smiled, "Yep, welcome to Iowa."

The strong northern wind was blasting through the state. It caused many snow pile-ups along the roads, over sidewalks, and over many parts of the interstate. My 4X4 truck plowed through them as if they were not even there.

The drive-up for valet parking at the Cancer Center was in high demand on cold days like this. Many cars were backed up onto the regular street. Several cars were parked along the sidewalk, and the consistent small puffs of warm vapor coming from their exhausts, clarified that they were still running. The two gentlemen that always have plenty of time to welcome you with a warm smile were now rushing around, from car to car, to get everyone in as soon as they could.

"I am going to park it myself in the garage, babe," I told Becky.

"Those guys are way too busy right now."

Becky was now holding her hands in front of the heater that was blowing hot air into the truck, warming her hands.

"Okay, honey," she said.

Although the parking garage was not heated, I was sure I would be able to find a parking spot close to one of the entrances that were located on every floor. From there, a heated walkway provided warmth and coverage from the parking garage to the hospital and clinics.

Since we had a handicapped sticker, parking close was not a problem. On the second floor, right next to the entrance to the walkway, I saw an empty parking spot as if it were designed for us. Four wheelchairs were conveniently parked right inside the building. From there, it was only a five-minute walk through the warm skywalk.

I rolled her wheelchair right next to an open seat in the waiting room of the oncology clinic. After I secured the brakes, I sat down next to her in one of the regular chairs. I brought my hand over to her lap and there, our fingers weaved together. Many people were there that day, so the waiting room was full. There were patients of all ages, some barely old enough to vote, too many in their mid-forties. Most of them showed concerning signs of illness, frail skin with a gray tone, skinny, and bald heads covered with hand knitted beanies. My eyes continued to travel past the many that were facing, or had already faced, the barbaric emotional rollercoaster of cancer.

I gazed past all the sickness, out the window, observing the frozen tundra outside, focusing on the two guys that were always there to help park your car. They would open the doors for any patient coming out of their vehicles, always lending a hand or an arm to lean on for those who were weak on their feet. They were always willing to run inside to grab a wheelchair and get you inside where you needed to be. I do not know why, but my thoughts were going out to them, realizing that they were always there to help, and that they were also faced with the sudden disappearance of patients.

I wondered if they also felt sadness, or even got emotional when they suddenly realized that someone was no longer coming back to the clinic. Did they ever wonder what happened to those patients? Did they talk amongst each other and ask 'what happened to so-and-so?' Did anyone ever talk to them about that?

I realized, just sitting there, gazing past all these sick people, past their life-absorbing cancer, that those two guys, the two older men, tried to make a difference by helping, smiling, lending a hand or an arm to lean on. How did they handle the pain and sadness of those not returning?

Angie came to take us back to the exam room before we went to the lab for bloodwork. At every appointment, lab work would be completed. Normally by the time we sat down and talked to Doctor Freeman, he would already have the results. Today everything just seemed out of place, more hectic and disorganized than normal.

"Don't worry about the labs right now," Angie explained.

"We will do those later."

She unlatched the brakes from the wheelchair and started to take Becky towards the exam rooms in the back of the clinic. The room, as always, was immaculate, clean, and well organized. Angie was positive and optimistic as always.

Doctor Freeman came in, smiling as usual. Today he seemed more cheerful than normal. After he sat down in the office chair that was parked at the desk, he turned towards us, leaning forward, both elbows resting on his knees. He had a big smile on his face, sparkling eyes like a boy that just got a Christmas present he asked for, almost triumphant. He jumped right into the facts.

"So, we got your MRI results back," he said, "and they show improvement at the locations of the leptomeningeal metastasis."

He pulled up the written report on the screen and pointed out the final impression from the radiologist at the bottom of the report. *'Improved leptomeningeal metastatic disease.'* While Freeman gave us the details, I felt Becky's hand tighten inside mine. I could feel the excitement flowing through her.

"So, it seems that the treatment is working?" she carefully asked.

He moved his attention from the computer screen to her, smiled, and responded as conservatively as possible.

"It seems that the current treatment is keeping things under control," he said, as he took a deep breath in and exhaled slowly.

The snow under my feet made a cracking sound. With every step I could feel it breaking under the rubber soles of my boots. My steps were rapidly increasing as I gained better control in anticipation of the slickness from the ice underneath the fresh fallen snow. My truck was in front of the emergency department entrance, alarm-blinkers on, to alert traffic of my position.

As the double sliding glass doors opened with a swift swoosh, I leaned through the opening to retrieve one of the wheelchairs that were conveniently parked just around the corner of the glass wall. The wheels were sliding through the snow, leaving curved tracks. My gloved hand reached the handle of the passenger door and a quick short jerk opened it.

Becky was staring at me with eyes that were screaming for help, her breathing rapid and shallow. I almost completely carried her from the seat of my truck to the wheelchair. The shortness of breath was so intense she could barely find the energy to contract her own muscles and support her own weight. I slammed the door shut and pushed towards the entrance of the emergency department. The snow combined with the previous ice-layer caused the wheels to have a mind of their own. The wheelchair seemed to go in the opposite direction I wanted it to go. By force I was able to push and turn it through the frozen resistance into the hospital.

Earlier that morning, after I had taken the boys to school, I arrived back home and made some coffee. As I scooped the freshly ground coffee from the small grinder into the filter, the aroma travelled through the air and my senses picked up the sweet bitter fragrance. At that moment I could not resist the,

"Ahh, that smells so good."

The sudden worrisome sound of my name coming from the bedroom triggered an immediate emergency response. Within seconds I arrived at our bedroom. Becky was sitting upright, both hands on the bed pushing herself up.

"I can't breathe," was all she could burst out.

Her breathing was rapid and shallow, her eyes stared straight forward, focused on nothing but her breathing. Immediately I reached out for the nebulizer and albuterol to give her a breathing treatment to open up her airway. It seemed to relieve the discomfort a little, but within an hour, she continued to have the same problems again. This time I tried to coach her through the episode, but soon I realized that it was not relieving the shortness of breath.

Even after another nebulizer treatment, her breathing continued to stay alarmingly fast. A visit to the emergency department was the only sensible option. Instead of waiting six minutes on the ambulance if I were to call 911, I determined that the fastest option was to drive her myself. After a hasty departure from our home, I called the charge nurse to inform her of my arrival and of the situation at hand. I was pleased to hear that Shari answered the phone. We had worked together many times and she was well aware of the situation with Becky.

"Just come through the main entrance," she said. "The garage is filled with ambulances right now."

I knew she would normally allow me to park in the ER garage, since it was so brutally cold outside.

"I will tell the front desk to just take you to room 7 immediately," she said.

"We will do the check in later."

I approached the front desk and the triage nurse recognized me from a distance. Without hesitation, she pushed the button underneath the counter to open the large heavy oversized door that would allow access to the ER. The triage nurse noticed the deteriorating state Becky was in, stood up, and followed us.

As we came through the door, Shari was sitting at her desk. She turned her head to see who was coming in. She was looking straight at us. Her eyes first aimed at me, then to Becky. The change of her facial expression revealed her concern. She instantly stood up, tapped on the window behind her, where most of the providers would be, and almost yelled,

"ER doc room 7 STAT!"

By the time I turned the corner to get into room 7, a barrage of medical personnel had arrived; two nurses, Shari, the triage nurse, and the ER doc. As they were helping Becky from the wheelchair onto the bed, I provided a rapid report with only the pertinent facts, just as I would do when delivering a patient to the ER with the ambulance. No personal stuff, no time for unimportant information. As they started to hook her up to the monitor, the ER doc was listening to Becky's lungs. After a short assessment of her lung sounds, he ordered,

"Chest X-ray STAT!"

He looked at Shari and confirmed,

"Diminished bilateral lung sounds. I want a non-rebreather at 15 liters!"

As I stood there, I was observing my team, my fellow nurses, in full alert mode taking care of my Becky. Normally I would be there helping them, as a fellow nurse and team member. Now I stood at the sidelines, as the spouse of a patient. I knew that she was in great hands, my team was the best, and although I wanted to help, I knew I would only be in the way.

Within minutes Becky was attached to every possible monitor: EKG, blood-pressure, and pulse-ox. She was receiving high-flow oxygen via a non-rebreather mask, blood was drawn, and radiology had just walked it with the portable X-ray machine.

The ER doc waived me to come over to look at the chest X-ray. Just outside Becky's room, the portable X-ray machine displayed the image of Becky's chest. It showed two large darkened areas behind both lungs.

"Just what I thought," he said, "fluid behind her lungs."

He turned towards one of the nurses and ordered,

"Get interventional radiology on the phone for me, please."

As the nurse walked away, he gestured me to follow him back into the room where Becky was. He explained to Becky that there was a lot of fluid on her lungs and that it would have to be drained via thoracentesis.

"Once the fluid is removed, you will be able to breathe normally again," he explained.

Since it would be best to do this under the guidance of an ultrasound, it would have to be done by interventional radiology.

"They will numb an area on your back," he explained to Becky, "and then they will insert a drain to remove all the fluid."

The procedure room was darkened. The machinery and screens used for the ultrasound images provided a strange greenish glow in the room. The air was cool, not cold, but low enough to notice the air flowing over your skin. The distinct hospital smell was present in this room. Becky was sitting on the edge of the bed. A large table was placed in front of her. She had placed both her arms on the table, hunched forward. She was wearing the usual blue hospital gown, but this time with the back open. Sterile drapes were taped to the skin of her back. The yellow color of Betadine indicated that the skin was properly prepped. I was standing right next to her. From there I could see what was happening and, more importantly, support Becky. I knew that this was going to be uncomfortable, but the reward of being able to breathe normally would be worth it.

The radiologist completed the initial imaging with the ultrasound to determine the best location to penetrate into the lung cavity. A syringe was prepared with a long large bore needle. It was purposefully placed on the metal table that was covered with a blue draping to indicate that the area was sterile.

Lidocaine was used to numb the area where the radiologist would insert the needle. Next to the syringe was a long plastic tube that would be attached to the needle to allow the fluid from Becky's lungs to be drained into empty plastic bottles. With the ultrasound in his left hand, placed on Becky's back, he observed the images on the screen, then he raised his right hand with his fingers and thumb open into a grabbing position,

"Lidocaine please."

The nurse placed the syringe in his hand, then removed the plastic cap from the needle. Right before he pushed the metal needle into Becky's skin, he warned her,

"Big stick here."

The needle slid into her skin with ease, and as he started to push the plunger forward to inject the lidocaine, the skin raised up a little. It turned a lighter color, almost white. Immediately Becky made a soft moaning sound, squeezed my hand, but did not move as he had instructed her earlier.

"This is the painful part," he said. "I am sorry."

He continued to increase the amount of the numbing agent under her skin, moving the needle deeper and deeper into her back to assure it would be completely numb. Every time he would advance a little deeper, Becky tightened her grip in my hand; I knew this was painful.

He placed the empty syringe back on the metal table, right next to the larger one with the large bore needle. As he let go of the smaller syringe, his fingers found the bigger one, and picked it up without deviating his attention from Becky's back. With the ultrasound still in his other hand that was securely placed on her skin, it continued to display pictures on the screen from Becky's lungs and where the fluid was. His eyes switched between Becky's back and the screen to make sure he advanced this large needle inside her lung cavity at the right location. Slowly he brought the large needle closer to her skin while he continued to scan between her skin and the screen.

"Big stick," he announced and without delay he advanced the large metal rod into her skin between the ribs. On the screen a large white stick represented the needle. He moved it up and down several times before he advanced the needle deeper into the darkened area in Becky's lung-cavity; that was where all the fluid was. Slowly he pulled on the plunger to create a vacuum to suck out the fluid and immediately the chamber of the syringe started to fill with a clear yellow liquid. As he put the ultrasound device down, the nurse handed him the tubing.

A small device between the hub of the needle and the syringe allowed him to turn on or off certain flow-ways. He attached the tubing to one of the tabs, removed the syringe, and as the nurse placed the other end of the tubing into the bottle, he opened the valve towards the drain. A rapid flow of yellowish fluid came out, filling up the 500 ml bottle within several minutes.

"Exchange bottles please," he requested the nurse.

The new bottle was placed, the flow continued, now at a much slower rate, but still consistent.

"Oh my God," Becky stated, "I can breathe again."

He explained to Becky that the fluid was still coming out but that they already filled a half-liter bottle. When the flow of the fluid slowed down to almost dripping, he reached for the ultrasound and tried to determine if all the fluid was gone.

"There might be a little fluid left," he said, "but it is very minimal."

He removed the needle and concluded the procedure. He placed gauze and tape over the puncture wound, then showed Becky both bottles that were almost full.

"We drained one liter of fluid from your lungs," he confirmed.

"We will send a sample to the lab to get it analyzed."

Becky, now sitting upright, was just happy that she was able to breath normally. She looked at me, smiled, her eyes shining bright.

"Doing much better now honey" she said.

Sixteen

The walls of the waiting room at the Hematology and Oncology office were once again staring back at us. Once a month we were contained within its grip and sometimes even more frequently than planned. The art pieces on the walls, the old magazines on the tables, and the plastic plants were all becoming too boring and too familiar. Several days ago, a 'restaging' CT-scan was completed to determine if there was any activity. In a couple of weeks, we also had an appointment for a new MRI of the neck and brain. Only an MRI could determine if there was any growth in the brain or neck area.

Angie came to get us to bring us back to the exam room. After she completed her assessment, she left to inform Doctor Freeman we were ready. Becky and I were, as usual, sitting next to each other, holding hands. We were both scared and excited at the same time; scared for the possibility of bad news, excited for the possibility of good news. Every time any imaging was completed, our unspoken fears and hopes would collide, but we always prayed for that miracle.

Doctor Freeman entered the room, and I noticed that his demeanor revealed some unhappiness. Although he tried to cover it up with his usual positive attitude, I picked up that something was bugging him. We discussed in detail the recent thoracentesis episode, and he explained that sometimes lung cancer can cause increased fluid production around the lungs.

"These episodes can be very sporadic or can become more chronic," he said.

"We will have to deal with them as they occur."

He explained that he was putting in 'a standard order' with the interventional radiology department, so if it happened again, we could go directly to them to get a thoracentesis done, and skip going to the ER.

He rolled his office chair towards the desk, typed his ID and password on the keyboard and brought the screen to life. As he turned the screen towards us, he gestured to us to move closer.

"Let me show you the images of the new CT scan," he told us.

Becky's CT scan appeared on the screen and as Freeman rolled the little wheel of his mouse up and down, the screen showed the different images. He froze on one image that showed the main tumor in her left upper lung. He opened another window on the screen and pulled up the CT scan from two months ago. He placed the two images next to each other for us to compare.

"As you can see here," using his pencil circling the area of concerns, "it seems that the primary tumor is growing."

The air became heavy. Silence revealed an unexpected numbness. Our eyes were focused on the screen, hoping for a mistake, but the obvious result was staring us straight in the face. I could feel Becky's silence screaming for help.

'How can this be? She was doing so much better. Why is this happening?' My mind tried to find a reason but returned empty handed.

Before Becky or I could respond, Doctor Freeman continued.

"It seems that it has grown about 1 centimeter in diameter."

He laid his pencil down, turned himself towards us so that he was facing us straight on.

"That is why you were probably having all that fluid build-up behind your lungs," he explained.

He informed us that instead of having to go and get a thoracentesis done every time there is fluid on the lungs, Becky could have a permanent valve placed in the chest to drain the fluid. If shortness of breath occurred, all we had to do was to open the valve and drain the fluid ourselves.

Becky and I looked at each other and, almost in sync, tilted our head to one side, our eyebrows frowning. Becky looked at Doctor Freeman, and said,

"Nah, I think I will hold off on that one." She wanted to wait and see before having another procedure done.

"Okay," he said smiling.

"No problem, but if you change your mind, just let me know."

He returned his focus on the growing tumor and provided us with possible options to deal with this devastating development. I remembered he educated us in one of our first meetings that cancer has a mind of its own. It does not play fair, and it will usually find a way around the treatment because it will continue to evolve and mutate its structure so that it can continue to grow. He explained that it seemed that the cancer mutated enough so that the Tarceva had less impact.

"I am afraid that if we start chemotherapy, your quality of life will diminish to almost nothing," he added, "but I believe that we should start with radiation to control the tumor's growth."

Becky looked at me, softly nodded, telling me that she agreed.

Doctor Freeman's position was always clear about his goals in regard to any treatment option. His focus was always to prolong life while maintaining quality of life.

"What good is it if we prolong your life, but it is miserable because you are in so much pain and discomfort?" was one of his statements.

Both Becky and I agreed with him about that from day one.

On a positive note, and Freeman was always on the lookout for that, he voiced his delight that Becky was doing so well on the *'pulse-dosing'* with Tarceva.

"Becky," he said, "keep in mind that four months ago I told you that you might have six weeks left to live, but yet, here we are."

Becky's hand squeezed mine softly. She looked at me with her beautiful green eyes and a small collection of tears sat in the corner and caused a shiny glitter. She smiled and filled the room with her radiant happiness. It was true, and he was right. This was also a moment to celebrate, despite the negative results of the CT scan. Sometimes we lost sight of the positives.

The weather started to change from cold, freezing, snowy days, to typical spring storms with lots of rain, thunder, and the possibility for tornados. It was early in the afternoon, the sun was still low in the sky, shooting strong light-rays over mother earth. Although the temperature outside was still chilly enough to warrant long-sleeved shirts or light jackets, the branches on the trees started to sprout little green buds.

Farmers emerged from their winter slumber and crawled out from their homes. Like vampires they raised their forearms to block the bright sunlight penetrating their eyes. Their tractors, most of them green-colored, emerged from their barns and started to prep their lands. Big clouds of dirt were visible for miles. Birds came back home, landing on the freshly plowed land to hunt for food. A few of our Dutch tulips that we'd planted many years ago started to break through the wet earthy layer around the big pine trees in the front yard.

Over the last several weeks we had been back to the interventional radiology at least every other week to drain fluids from Becky's lungs. The fact that we were now able to just call Freeman's office and get a straight referral to that department made it much easier for us, since we didn't have to go through the emergency department every time.

Becky had her MRI restaging completed of her neck and brain. She was able to sit through the whole procedure without any issues. She managed to suppress her fear for small spaces. The results were astounding; her leptomeningeal disease was no longer detectable, and her brain tumors were dormant. The *'pulse-dosing'* with Tarceva seemed to suppress the cancer in her neck, and the radiation seemed to stagnate the growth in her brain.

Despite this positive news, Becky's pain continued to increase. More frequently she required stronger pain medicine to control her discomfort. We tried to convince Doctor Freeman to allow Becky to have a PCA, but in his professional opinion he would only go that route when a patient was in hospice, facing the final steps of life.

***

The bedroom was filled with chatter, Lisa was visiting Becky. Their voices travelled through the hallway into the kitchen where I was rinsing off the dishes from last night's dinner and putting them in the dishwasher. Their voices sometimes loud, then soft, followed by laughter and some episodes of silence. I knew that in those moments of stillness both Lisa and Becky would be wiping away tears.

I squirted the liquid dishwasher soap into the slot on the inside of the dishwasher door. A loud click confirmed that the door was closed. I pushed *'normal wash'* followed by *'start.'* Immediately a soft, but noticeable whooshing sound arose from the dishwasher, confirming the start of the washing cycle. My bare feet did not make any noise on the hardwood floor as I walked through the hallway towards our bedroom. Becky's and Lisa's voices became louder and clearer as I moved closer. I could hear they were talking about Connor and Dane.

The bedroom door was wide open, and our dog, Mondavi, was laying on the feet-end of our bed. Our cat was comfortably sleeping on top of Becky's pillow. Although it was our cat, Becky determined it was my cat since it would always bite everyone but me. I classified her biting more as a loving *'nibble'* as she had never broken anyone's skin or drawn blood...yet.

Our cat's name was Zinfandel, but everyone just called her Kitty. She received the name Zinfandel because of the color of her fur, a soft red, like a Zinfandel wine. You might have noticed that both of our animals were blessed with names of wines. This was a Becky thing; all her animals she ever had were named according to a type of wine or vineyard. Becky was an avid wine drinker, and her favorite wine was a red one that would *"Suck the moist out of your tongue,"* she would always say.

Her previous dog's name was Chablis and our previous cat's name was Asti. The interesting story about Zinfandel, our current cat, was that she and Becky did not really get along well. Becky would always avoid her and vice versa. I knew the feeling was mutual because they would walk in large circles around each other. However, it was amazing to notice that from the moment Becky was diagnosed with lung cancer, the cat suddenly decided to sleep with her every moment of the day. She would not just position herself somewhere on the bed, oh no, she would place herself on top of Becky's pillow, wrap her body around Becky's head, and just snore away.

It freaked Becky out because she did not understand the sudden affection. Later, she explained that she read an article that cats can sense when a person is dying and that they will lay with them. You may be wondering why I am telling you all this about our pets. Any person that has pets knows that they are important family members and that they can sense emotions. They know when you are sad, they know when you are happy.

To Becky, her dog was very important. Mondavi was already seventeen years old and had been with Becky since he was a puppy. Mondavi would always sit with Becky, follow her around, and always lay on the bed with us.

Both animals were present on the bed and Becky was sitting upright. Lisa was sitting on the far side of the bed. When I walked into the bedroom, both their heads turned to me and as expected, I saw four red eyes; they had been crying and that was ok.

After I planted a quick kiss on Becky's lips, I sat down at the foot end of the bed, right next to Mondavi.

"What are you girls talking about?" I asked.

"Oh, just nothing and everything," Becky answered.

"Mhm," I sarcastically responded.

I knew very well that they were talking about emotional issues. As if the red eyes and the wad of tissues on the bed did not give away anything.

As I tried to mingle into the conversation, Becky suddenly raised her hands, opening and closing them simultaneously, gesturing that she wanted me to come over to her. I was assuming she wanted a hug or a kiss.

I raised up from the bed and within two steps I was right by her side. Instead of widening her arms for a hug, she narrowed the space between her hands and entrapped my face by cupping both her hands around it. She pulled me close to her face and her eyes began to water. Suddenly gentle tears were released and rolled softly down her cheeks. Her voice dropped to a whisper; a delicate shiver underlined her words. As she spoke, she shook my head a little up and down, to make sure I was paying attention.

"Honey," she started.

"Yes?" as she had my undivided attention.

"I don't think that I am going to make it."

My eyes stung, gentle tears were building up and trying to escape. I tried to hold back, clenching my jaws together causing the muscles along my face to contract. I did not say anything.

"I don't think I can beat this one," she continued.

I was drowning in her pupils.

"You have to promise me that you will take care of my boys, because if you don't, I will come down to haunt you," she emphasized.

I could no longer restrain my emotions, the tears now freely running down my face falling into her lap. She used her thumb to wipe them away. My heart was breaking, being ripped out of my chest. Our souls flowing together as one, all other things faded, with perfect silence.

She had to say it, she had to get it off her chest. It was laying as a heavy load on her shoulders that she could no longer bear to carry. It felt like a knife cutting deep in my chest and leaving gaping bleeding wounds that were beyond repair. She let go of my face, I leaned forward and as our arms pulled our bodies closer, we both broke down. Tears were running down our faces, our bodies shivering, our shoulders shrugging. My lips released a soft whisper.

"I love you honey."

Our kiss confirmed our understanding and our commitment.

A beautiful spring evening invited us to sit outside. The amazing scent released by trees, plants, and flowers was unique on its own. Fresh air was flowing with a soft gentle breeze, cooling down one of the first nice warm and dry days of spring. The moon was still asleep, but many stars were sparkling brighter than ever. Living out in the country seemed to intensify the brightness of the nightly presentation of faraway galaxies, planets, and stars. Both boys were asleep, resting for an early morning awakening to enjoy another day of school. Our eyes were attracted to the beautiful display of the stars. We were slouched on the wicker loveseat with Becky laying in my arms.

"Do you remember?" she softly spoke.

The moment she spoke, I knew exactly what she was talking about.

"Oh yeah babe," I said, "I remember."

It was summer of 1998. Although I still had my apartment, I would spend most of my time at her townhome. Frequently at night, if the weather was nice, she would grab a big blanket, place it on the grass, and with a glass of wine in our hands, we would snuggle together and just stare at the beautiful skies. We tried to find shooting stars or discover a very bright one, or maybe a new galaxy. We would lay there for hours, not saying much, just enjoying the beautiful evening in each other's arms. Tonight, we did just that.

Serenity creates peace and harmony. Words sometimes ruin the moments. Silence allows inner peace and thoughts.

"You know honey," Becky suddenly said after being soaked in this perfect stillness for almost an hour, her voice soft and calm.

"We have been through a lot, people have tried to bring us down, and people will continue to do so, even after I am gone."

My breathing became shallow, my heart pounding. It hurts when she was so painfully honest. I tightened my grip on her, closing our bodies together.

"I want you to write our story," she continued. "I want you to let the world know what we have been through."

My hand in hers, her thumb gently stroking the back of my hand, my face next to hers, smelling her intoxicating essence, I closed my eyes as my breathing became deep and slow. I sensed her smell, the softness of her skin, the sweet taste of her lips, and the radiant beauty of her soul.

"The world needs to know what we have been through," she said, confirming her devotion.

"Okay honey, I will," I responded and sealed the promise with a kiss.

Wednesdays were my work days. Once a week I would work a twelve-hour shift at the ER. It provided me with a little break from everything. Just one day a week I could focus my mind on something else. On these days, Becky's sister would come over to take care of Becky and our boys. Although a normal shift would start at 7am, I requested a later start, at 8am, so that I could take the boys to school.

I pulled up at Dane's school and, as usual, cars were in a long line to drop kids off at the front entrance of the building. It was a beautiful spring day and I decided to park my truck behind the church that was across the street. Dane was all chatter when I turned onto the parking lot. As I got out of the truck, the fresh, crisp, spring air aroused my senses. The invigorating morning scent had a unique bouquet of aromas from the early morning dew that was clinging on to the grass blades. I took a deep breath in through my nose to draw in more of that morning spring fragrance.

Dane jumped out of the truck as if he had been trapped in there for centuries. His backpack hanging from one shoulder, his bright blond hair long and waving in the wind. His hand immediately grabbed mine, and while we walked towards the school, he was unable to stop talking. Out of the blue he suddenly mentioned something about a school performance.

"What performance are you talking about buddy?" I asked since I was unaware of anything. Normally the school would insert flyers or send emails about these events. I could have overlooked it, not noticed it or tossed it in the trash.

"The singing performance this morning!" he answered.

"What?!" I responded confused.

"You have a performance this morning?"

"Yeah, we have been practicing for weeks" he said, "and it is at ten this morning."

Damn.

"I didn't know that Dane. You should have told me so I could have taken time off from work."

"I thought you knew, Papa," he said with a sad face.

I knew he was upset because we would normally never miss anything from school. While I was holding Dane's hand and we were walking towards the school, I called Lisa to see if she was working. I knew that if at least someone would show up, he would feel better.

"Hey, what's up?" Lisa answered.

I started to explain the situation, asking her if she could come over to see Dane's performance.

"Absolutely", she responded without hesitation.

"I am not working today, so I will be there at ten."

She also said that she would bring her iPad to record the performance so Becky could see it later that day.

"Awesome," I said.

"I will let Dane and Becky know."

At the front entrance of the elementary school, there were two large wooden doors. Both were wide open, and each side was guarded by a teacher. Parents were allowed to bring their kids into the school, but no strangers had access. All these security measures came in place after all the school shootings.

The school principal smiled and waved.

"Good morning Dane, good morning Mister Slootheer."

The hallways were chaotic, as children were running all over, with loud voices, some screaming, while parents were dropping their kids off at their classrooms. On the walls were hooks with name-tags above them. I leaned over towards Dane while dodging running kids and explained that Lisa would be coming to see his performance and that she would record it so Mama and I could see it later.

His bright smile with glistening eyes and his exclamation of,

"Yay, Lisa is coming!" explained how he felt about that.

I was just glad that someone was able to come and see Dane perform.

I waved goodbye to the school principal that was still standing at the door receiving young wild humans into the building. As I walked towards my truck, my mind was searching through my memories trying to remember if I missed anything about his performance. I did not remember hearing or seeing anything about it.

I had to hurry, since I had to be at work in twenty minutes and it was at least a fifteen-minute drive. I left the parking lot, turning onto the main street through our little town that would lead to the interstate.

I glanced at my watch and shook my head. *I am never going to make it on time.*

I browsed through my contacts on my phone for 'charge nurse ER.' I knew I was going to be late and I needed to let them know. The phone rang twice, and a female voice answered,

"Mercy ER charge nurse."

"Hey, this is Roy. I am running a little late," I said.

"That's okay," she said, "we are at a low census anyway right now."

I realized that, since it was a low census, I could just ask if I could come in later so I could go see Dane's performance.

"Sure, no problem," she responded, "just get here around noon, ok?"

"Great! Thank you! My son will be very happy to see me there," I told her.

I had almost arrived at the interstate but made a quick U-turn and started to drive back to Dane's school. I called Becky to inform her about the recent developments from this morning.

"Hey babe, it's me," I said when she answered the phone.

"It seems that Dane has a performance this morning. Did you know about that?" I asked her.

Becky was also unaware of anything going on at the school. I told her that I could take time off from work to go see him and that Lisa would also come to the school, and that she would record it on her iPad.

"I am sure that she will stop by after," I told her, "so you can see it too, sweetie."

After we were done talking, I called Lisa to let her know I was coming after all.

"Can you save me a spot," I asked her.

"Of course," she responded.

The small school gym was packed with parents and other kids. They placed the stadium seating benches along the far wall to allow more people to be able to sit. Most kids were sitting in front of the stadium-seating on the ground, close to the stage. Teachers were strategically positioned around the stage and by all the doors. The chatter was loud and overwhelming. I tried to find Lisa in the crowd. Suddenly I noticed her standing up and raising her hand, waving. She was sitting on the highest row, all the way to the left.

Trying to make my way up there was a challenge, people were not respecting the walkways between the benches, and kids and adults were just sitting wherever they could. As I stepped over legs, squeezed through bodies, avoided heads and tried not to twist an ankle on my mission to the top, I made it without scratches or bruises. Lisa welcomed me with a big hug. Lisa, I must say, is a great hugger. You can feel her warm heart and true genuine care and love through these hugs. We sat and talked until the show started.

After the performance was over, I decided to stop by the house before heading out to work. Since I was still in town, I just wanted to give my sweet Becky another kiss and hug. At that time, I did not realize the disaster I was about to walk into.

I pulled up to the house. It was a gorgeous spring day with blue skies, small clouds like little puffs sporadically placed here and there, with a perfect temperature of the mid-70s. The dew drops from this morning that were clinging onto the grass blades had disappeared and left them bright green and intense. I assumed that Becky would be sitting on the deck in the back of the house, enjoying a cup of tea and this beautiful day.

When I came through the front door, I noticed suppressed sounds travelling through the hallway. Surprised, since I was expecting them to be outside, I walked to our bedroom. There I was met by four red eyes with swollen eyelids staring at me. Something had happened here, something bad, something that made them both cry.

"What's going on here?" I asked confused.

Both very much upset and emotional. Becky explained that we had another family disaster earlier that morning. Once again, Becky was confronted by a family member that was unable to control stress, frustration, fear, and anger. This time, this person attacked Becky. It was difficult enough for her to deal with her own cancer, but now she was forced to also deal with the explosive outburst from someone else.

For any of you who are reading this story, keep in mind that if you ever get exposed to a similar situation, or already have been, it is important to realize that most these aggressive outbursts are not aimed at any person, it is just the frustration towards the situation.

I held Becky in my arms. She was shivering from pain, as if she had just come out of a blistering cold winter storm. We sat there, together on the bed, holding each other like wounded soldiers on a battlefield that were thrown into an unwanted war caused by the betrayal by one of our own. Now we were not only dealing with the physical wounds of the attack, but also the emotional impact of such treason.

Seventeen

"I really think you will benefit from some assistance, Roy," Angie said.

"I agree," Becky said, supporting her, "I think Angie has a good point."

"Ok, I guess we can give it a try," I responded reluctantly, since I was not sure I wanted to do this.

We were discussing the possibility of utilizing home-health-nursing. This is when a nurse comes to your home several times a week to help out with basic medical care. The initial plan was to have them come over three times a week to check vital signs and access Becky's port to make sure it was still functioning properly. They would also administer any medications, if needed.

Becky continued to have increased episodes of severe pain, shortness of breath, coughing, nausea, and diarrhea mixed with episodes of constipation. Frequently, we had to run to the ER to get further care. Our fridge started to look like a private pharmacy, and since Becky had a port, I administered most of her medicine intravenously. Zofran, Phenergan, Ativan, and Alprazolam were just a few that I had available at home to manage complications. Since pain was the main issue, liquid Morphine was recently added to our supplies.

During the last visit we had with Doctor Freeman, I provided him with a new research article that I found in the *'Journal for Clinical Oncology.'* This research study discussed the benefit of adding Avastin to the treatment of Tarceva.

Avastin is a medicine that blocks the growth of new blood-vessels, and since cancer needs more nutrition as it grows, it seeks to create new blood vessels to increase blood supply to the tumor. Avastin would block such development, and as the growth of blood vessels becomes restricted, blood supply would not get to the tumor and thus it would starve. Avastin was the same medicine that was injected into Becky's eye, and we saw that tumor completely disappear. This study showed improvement in patients with the combination of Tarceva and Avastin. Doctor Freeman wanted to do some more research on his own before making a recommendation.

It had been almost a year since we first came into the Hematology and Oncology clinic where we met with Doctor Freeman and his nurse Angie. I had the feeling we were more than just patients. We talked about many things and, since Angie was a single mom with three boys, we shared a lot of fun, sad, and bad experiences we had as parents. During one of our visits, Angie suddenly asked,

"So how did you guys meet?"

"The old-fashioned way, in a bar," was my immediate response.

"Yep, no internet involved with us," Becky confirmed with a big smile.

As we continued to talk about how we met, Becky leaned forward, placed her hand on Angie's knee, and while giggling she said,

"Let me tell you how we decided to get married...."

"We talked about getting married at a certain point in time, but I did not decide one way or the other," Becky said as she started to lean back in her seat.

I knew the story that was coming, it was quite funny, so I just observed my sweetheart glow with happiness as she shared this moment with Angie.

"So, Roy was at the grocery store picking up stuff for dinner and I was home, doing I don't know what."

Becky had this smirk on her face you'd see when one of your kids is doing something that they were not supposed to be doing. Her eyes were bright and filled with joy and menace.

"And while I was just sitting at home, thinking about that issue of marriage," she paused to take a deep breath.

"I decided I wanted to marry this man. He brought me joy and love and the fact that he actually made me wonder about marrying him was reason enough for me to do so."

She looked at me with those irresistible eyes, from which no escape was possible. She puckered her lips and blew me a kiss. I smiled.

"So, I called him to tell him we needed something else from the store, and while I was talking to him, adding items to the grocery list, I told him that I thought we should go ahead and get married."

"His response was hilarious," Becky exclaimed with laughter.

He said, "Ehhhh, are you asking me to marry you?"

"I guess," Becky said.

"I could hear Roy cracking up on the other side of the line and he said,

"So, while I am shopping at a grocery store, you are proposing to me! Wow, that's romantic!" and he could not stop laughing."

Both Angie and Becky were laughing out loud. Tears were rolling down their cheeks. My heart jumped and was filled with happiness to see my sweetheart laughing like that.

Lisa's car was in the driveway. She picked up the boys from school since we had our appointment with Doctor Freeman. Becky was getting more fatigued by the day. Even with the slightest activity, she needed to rest afterwards. The trip to Doctor Freeman's clinic and all the excitement of sharing stories with Angie had worn her out. I walked around the truck to open her door and as I wrapped one of my arms around her, I placed the other in front of her as support for her to lean on. She confessed,

"Oh my God honey, I am so tired."

"I know babe," I responded.

"Let's get upstairs and I will get you in bed so you can take a nap, okay?"

As we walked towards the front door, she placed both her hands on my arm that was in front of her. My other arm was around her, holding her close to me. I left the passenger door of the truck open. I would get that later. She was so fatigued that my focus was solely on getting her upstairs and into our bed.

Her increased weakness was troubling me. I believed it was a sign that the cancer was eating away her energy again, even though most of the scans showed she was actually doing better. The leptomeningeal disease was, as far we knew, no longer there and the main tumor in her left lung had stopped growing. I was afraid it had spread all over her body, but that it was still too small to detect.

I never stopped my research. Daily I climbed behind my laptop, when everyone was asleep, trying to find new discoveries about cancer treatments, or upcoming new developments. I continued to make Becky juices, cook organic foods and tried to stay within the diet according to Doctor Moerman's recommendations. Deep inside me, deep down in my gut, I was scared, I was worried, I was afraid, but I never showed that to anyone. I could not show my fears, I had to stay positive, I had to stay strong for Becky and our boys.

Becky was sitting on the edge of the bed. Her breathing was shallow and rapid. Her hands were on the bed supporting herself, trying to stay upright. Just from getting from the truck to the bed had completely worn her out. As I removed her clothes, I stayed aware of her position since I was afraid that she might fall over.

After I undressed her, I put on her favorite fleece pajamas. I remembered she'd asked me to buy some of those for her, so I bought five pairs of them. I helped her lie down in bed. She immediately rolled onto her right side and curled up. I pulled the comforter up over her shoulder. With delicate precision, I placed my hand on her cheek, leaned forward, and kissed her lips.

"I Love you honey," I said.

Her eyes glittered with tears; she was worried. I knew she was scared too.

"Get some rest, ok?" I confirmed.

"Ok babe. Love you," she said as she closed her eyes slowly.

Lisa was sitting outside on the deck, facing the back yard where the boys were running around, dragging all kinds of pieces of wood, sticks and other things towards the big old oak tree. The sliding door made a soft but noticeable noise to alert Lisa of my arrival.

"Hey," she said softly, "where is Beck?"

"I just put her in bed, she was worn out," I explained as I closed the sliding door.

Lisa smiled, stood up, and opened her arms to welcome a hug.

"Thank you for taking care of Connor and Dane," I said as my arms wrapped around her.

"No worries," she responded. "I love taking care of those boys."

We both sat down.

"What are they doing?" I asked Lisa.

"I have no clue," she said, "but it seems they are on a mission."

"That's obvious," I said laughing.

Lisa asked about the visit with Doctor Freeman. I told her about the discussion I had with him in regard to the research I found about the benefits of using Avastin in combination with Tarceva. I also explained that Angie was promoting home healthcare, and that Doctor Freeman's office would apply for this. Hopefully, someone from that organization would get a hold of me this week to discuss the details.

When the boys noticed I was sitting on the deck, they came running towards me, flew into my arms, and many kisses were exchanged. They never had many questions about how things were, or what was going on. They trusted me that I would tell them. Most of the time we talked at night while we sat in front of the TV. The boys would ask questions, or we would tell them about whatever was important enough for them to know.

"So, what are you guys building down there?" I asked, because I was still curious.

"A zombie fort," they both exclaimed!

"Another zombie fort?" I asked confused.

"Have you seen that TV show *'The Living Dead'*?" Connor asked.

"Nope," I honestly responded.

"Well, it is awesome!" Dane exclaimed.

"And with our forts we can keep the zombies out!" Connor added.

They both jumped up, grabbed my hand and dragged me over to their contraption. As they pulled me along, Lisa stood up, smiled and told me that she would check on Becky. Both boys showed me with pride the sticks in the ground pointing outwards that were supposed to spear zombies if they tried to attack them. A part of a metal fence, spiked to the ground, would cause electrocution of zombies if they stepped on it, and strings with cans attached would function as an alarm for them to know the zombies had arrived. All this was positioned around the old oak tree, since that was their base. It was amazing and fun to see the imagination they had.

The boys continued their imaginary war with the undead. Lisa was still gone. I decided to check on her and Becky. As I entered the hallway, I heard them talking. The door was open. Lisa was sitting on Becky's side, at her feet. It was obvious they were talking about cancer, disease, and death. Becky suddenly turned herself towards me, fear in her eyes, her hands shaking. She grabbed my face, her eyes staring straight at me, piercing through my soul. Tears started to collect in the corners of her eyes, her lips moved, her voice filled with fear.

"Honey, please don't let me die."

The words, although spoken softly, shouted painfully loud at me. She was so afraid. She counted on me and completely trusted me. Those words were engraved into my heart with a sharp tool, painfully etched onto my soul. Those words, "don't let me die", were heavy and loaded and would haunt me for the rest of my existence. My heart sunk into the deepest depths of my soul, screaming, shivering, alone in the dark night. The realization of complete failure, the feeling of powerlessness, paralyzed me. I was suddenly aware that I was incapable of changing what might be coming. With tears rolling down my face, I told her honestly,

"Oh honey, I am doing whatever I can do to prevent that."

The beautiful change of the seasons, from winter to spring, comes with a price in Iowa: storms. We had many of them with heavy downpours and tornadic activity. Frequently the tornado alarms would sound, and we all had to huddle down in the basement of the house to find shelter.

The boys were still up, but it was getting unusually early dark outside. The weatherman predicted severe storms throughout the evening and into the night. Not that we would ever really pay attention to his prediction, since he was wrong most of the time, but tonight seemed to be one of those nights he may actually have been right. The wind picked up after the sun settled for the day. Dark clouds lurked from high above and rolled into the area. They promised an increased chance for some massive rain.

Before the storm hit us, I decided to let Mondavi (our dog) go out. He was old and didn't want to walk far anymore, so we just let him out in the backyard. He would roam around the deck, do his business, and come back in.

I stood by the sliding door and called his name,

"Mondavi, let's go outside."

He appeared within minutes. Slowly he walked over to me, then sat down in front of the door.

"Let's go potty," I said as I opened it.

He walked onto the deck, tippled off the stairs into the grass and to the right of the deck. As usual he took a right turn, around the backside of the deck and disappeared out of view. While he was outside, I started to get the boys ready for bed.

"Ok guys, let's go take a shower."

"I will go first," Connor said as he jumped off the couch.

Dane continued to watch TV while Connor was showering. Meanwhile, I walked over to their bedroom to get some pajamas ready for them and placed them on the counter in the bathroom.

It must have been about ten minutes later when I decided to see if Mondavi was ready to come back in. Normally, he would be sitting in front of the sliding door to come back in, but when I glanced through the glass of the door, he was not there.

That's weird.

I opened the door, looked left, looked right. Maybe he was sitting somewhere on the deck, but he was not there.

"Mondavi," I yelled, "come here buddy."

Pouting my lips, I whistled several times. No response. I walked over to Dane and asked him,

"Did you let Mondavi in?"

His focus was still on the TV, he responded with a clear "No."

I walked to our bedroom. Becky was sitting in bed, reading.

"Did you let Mondavi back in honey?" I asked.

"No babe. Where is he?" as she raised her eyes from the pages and looked at me.

"I let him go out to potty," I explained, "but he is not back yet."

"He is probably just roaming around and digging something up," she said as she waved her hand in the air. She was probably right.

"Ok, I will take care of the boys first," I said.

Both boys were showered, teeth brushed, pajamas on, and they were now sitting on the couch until it was 8:30 PM. Mondavi was still outside. It must have been about 20 minutes since I let him go out, and I was getting really concerned at this time. Becky also expressed her worry.

"That's weird," she said.

She walked over to the window of our bedroom and opened it. She called his name several times.

"I think I can hear him, over there," she pointed towards the neighbor's house.

"Ok, I will go check," I said and started to make my way towards the back door.

I grabbed a light jacket as I passed the coat closet in the hallway, since the incoming storm had caused an impressive drop in temperature outside.

"Guys, I am going outside trying to find Mondavi," I said as I walked past them.

"You guys stay right here, okay?"

"Okay Papa," they both yelled, with their eyes still attached to the TV.

Once outside, I made my way over towards the direction Becky thought she could hear him. There were two rows of pine trees along the north side of the house, windbreakers they call them, because they helped to keep the cold northern winds off of the house. I thought maybe he had gotten stuck in there somewhere. On my way over I kept calling his name,

"Mondavi! Mondavi!"

I turned around the corner of the house, on the north side. Our bedroom window was open and Becky was hanging out from it. Before I could say anything, big fat raindrops started to come down. The initial release was slow. Becky yelled from the room,

"Over there babe," while she pointed towards the neighbor's house.

"I think I can hear him, but I don't see him!"

Before I could make my way around the pine trees, mother nature released a massive downpour. Within seconds I was hosed, completely soaked. My jacket, T-shirt, jeans, and shoes were all drenched. Regardless, I continued on my mission to find Mondavi. I roamed along the fence line, then climbed over it into the neighbor's yard, but Mondavi was nowhere to be found. The intensity of the rain decreased vision and sound to almost zero. The amount of water that was coming down was so intense, and combined with the poor lighting outside, I could see almost nothing.

I decided to use the headlights from my truck for illumination. I positioned myself under our bedroom, from where Becky was calling directions earlier. As I stood there, looking up, my eyelids blinking faster and faster trying to stave off the heavy raindrops, I placed my hand in front of my face as a shield. I called Becky's name several times before the window opened. It almost looked like a scene from Romeo and Juliet.

"Tell the boys to bring my keys to the front door!" I yelled.

The downpour was getting worse. Sound and sight were absorbed into the excessive rainfall. At this point in time I no longer tried to avoid the rain, even my underwear was drenched. I walked over to the front door. Connor was standing inside with my keys in his hand. As soon as he saw me getting closer, he opened it.

"Here are your keys Papa" he said. "You know you are all wet, right?"

Funny how kids like to bring the obvious to your attention.

"Yes, I know sweetie," I smiled, grabbed the keys and jumped in my truck.

My wet hands were resting on top of the steering wheel and water was running down my forearms. Streams of rain onto the rubber mats on the floor of my truck. My face was overrun with rainwater dripping from my soggy wet hair. I turned the ignition key and the engine came to life. The front windshield instantly started to fog up. As soon as I turned the air to *'defog'* it cleared rapidly.

I aimed my headlights into the field north of the house, just past the first section of pine trees. At first, I was planning to drive out there, but it was a steep downhill area and I noticed the rain started to form a pond at the bottom of the hill. I decided it was smarter just to leave the truck on the asphalt and not get it stuck in the mud. I aimed the headlights into the field. I voluntarily jumped back into the monsoon.

The pool of water at the bottom of the hill was about a foot deep. As I waded through the river, now halfway up my shins, my feet sank deep into the muddy dirt. My truck would have gotten stuck in this fast, even though it had four-wheel drive. I kept moving towards the far end, behind the pine trees. Becky was still at the window, but she could no longer hear Mondavi.

I decided to make a pass along the pine trees to see if I could find him. If not, he might have walked off somewhere else to hide from the rain. There were many spots he could have been, including our own barn or the one from the neighbors. I continued to call his name.

"Mondavi! Here boy!" I yelled in all directions.

"Mondavi!" But no response.

I did not hear or see anything. My headlights only reached about half-way down the pine trees; the rest remained in complete darkness. After another fifteen minutes of water peddling, I did not find him. I moved closer to our bedroom window where Becky still was standing, and I howled at her from a distance,

"I am going to drive up and down the road to see if he just took off!"

"Good idea!" she yelled back.

When I opened my truck door, I noticed that my seat had a wet outline of my body where I sat before. I jumped in the seat, making it more wet, and drove towards the road. First, I took a left turn, downhill. I turned my high beams on to improve the illumination of the road, the ditches, and the grass fields. I was hoping I would find him soon, as the weather was getting worse by the minute.

I drove five minutes one way, to the north, then turned around, drove ten minutes the other way, to the south. Then turned around and went back up the road again. Three times I made that loop, every time I went a little further down the road. After almost one hour of searching, I knew I was not going to be able to find him. He was not walking along the road.

Defeated, I parked the truck back into the driveway, when I suddenly thought of our back porch.

Maybe he is hiding under the porch?

The heavy spring storm welcomed me back outside as I walked around the back of the house and went down onto my knees to look under the wooden beams that supported the deck. It was a wide-open area that would have been a great hiding place for a stubborn little Bichon Frise like Mondavi. But no, nothing. I crawled through the mud towards the other side while I continued to call his name.

"Mondavi! Mondavi!" But no response.

Like a beaten dog, I walked back onto the deck. Saddened like a warrior that had just lost a battle, I knocked on the sliding door that was, as instructed by me earlier, locked by one of the boys. Becky appeared in my view. She had decided to get out of bed. She looked at me almost giggling. I must have looked horrible; soaked clothing, drenched hair, mud on my hands and knees, and I am sure it was somewhere on my face too. She tried to be sensitive and not to laugh, but I recognized that smirk that was the pre-runner for a total and complete outburst of laughter.

"Oh honey," she said with a smile, "come in, but let me get you a towel."

Both boys came flying around the corner, and when they saw me, they both cracked-up loudly. I could not help but smile. After my cleanup, Becky and I were sitting in our bed, the boys asleep. Becky had put them to bed while I was showering off my battle dirt.

"He is just hiding somewhere from the rain," Becky said.

Although I agreed with her, I still did not like him not being home.

The song of some early morning birds woke me up. The sun was already out, trying to peek through the crack of the curtains. I looked to my left to find Becky still asleep. For a moment, I lay there not thinking about anything. For a moment I even forgot what happened yesterday. Then suddenly, as if someone hit me with a hammer, I became aware of Mondavi not being here. I tried to roll over to my side as quietly as possible, so I could silently move out of the bed, but before I reached the edge and tried to escape from underneath the comforter, a soft,

"Good morning sweetie," came from Becky's side.

"Hey, you are awake," I surprisingly responded.

"Just now," she told me smilingly. "Where are you going?"

"To see if Mondavi is back," I replied.

I found him behind the pine trees in the far back of the neighbor's yard, the area where my headlights did not reach. He had gotten stuck in a net that was spread across the ground. Our neighbor had seeded that area with new grass and covered it with a special type of netting to prevent the wind from blowing the seeds away, or birds eating them, and to keep the moisture contained. When Mondavi walked over it, his little paws got stuck in the small holes of the netting. He must have fallen over and could not get back up. He had laid there all night, in the brutal spring storm with the massive downpours and cold wind.

When I found him, he was hyperventilating, unresponsive, shivering, and his little body was freezing cold. I cut the netting from around his paws, held him in my arms close to my body, trying to transfer some of my body heat to him. Becky saw me walking towards the house with his beaten little body in my arms.

"Is he okay?" she asked when I stepped into the house.

"I don't know sugar," I said, "he is not responding."

Becky wrapped a small blanket around him and grabbed him from my arms.

"If we would have had a working flashlight in the house, I would have found him yesterday," I said upset.

Becky placed him in his own soft warm and fluffy bed, covered him with another blanket trying to warm him up. I grabbed one of the syringes we had at home and tried to feed him a little water. But every time I would squirt a little in his mouth on one side, it would drip out on the other side. He was not doing well, but we were hopeful that if he warmed up, he would get better. After three hours there was no improvement. He was still unresponsive and shivering.

"I am taking him to the vet," I said.

The waiting room was still, except for two people, both with cats. They were both making loud wailing sounds, as if they were being tortured. It seemed they were competing against each other as they would alternate the howling. I had rolled Mondavi in his blanket like a burrito, and held him in my arms like a newborn, trying to warm his shivering body. On my way over to the vet hospital, I called ahead to let them know I was on my way. Becky wanted to come with me since Mondavi was her dog, but she was not feeling up to it. She did not have the energy to go.

The assistant came out within minutes of my arrival and placed us in a room. After he completed the intake and assessment, he said,

"The veterinarian will be with you shortly," and left through the opposite door from where we came in.

A steel tall table was standing in the middle of the room. On the counter there were some small plastic jars next to the faucet and a soap dispenser. A rubber mat was on the floor, along with some cabinets with closed doors. Besides that, the room was pretty much empty. A soft knock on the door and an older lady with dark gray hair, highlighted with bright white streaks, walked in. She had a kind face that was blessed with a genuine smile. After she introduced herself, I explained what had happened overnight. While she examined Mondavi, she said,

"Wow, I am shocked to know that he is seventeen years old." She looked up at me, "That's really old for these kinds of dogs."

"I know," I said as I nodded and smiled at her.

"I want to run some tests on him, but I will have to take him with me to the back. It will take about 30 minutes or so. Are you okay with that?" she asked.

"Yeah, that is fine," I responded.

While she was gone, I called Becky to give her an update about what was going on. I was still talking to her when the veterinarian walked back into the room.

"Gotta go babe," I said, "the vet just walked back in."

"Okay," Becky said, "call me back when you know more."

She told me that Mondavi was not doing well. Besides the fact that he seemed to be diabetic, his kidneys received a massive blow last night and they were both shutting down. She clarified that,

"Even if we get him better over the next several days, it is just a matter of time before his kidneys will completely fail and that would cause a horrible death."

We discussed the pros and cons of trying to save him. I asked her, "What would you do if Mondavi was your dog?"

"Although it would be a difficult decision for me," she said, "I would put him to sleep now, so he does not have to be in a lot of pain."

"I want to talk to my wife about this for a little," I said.

"Absolutely, I will be back in about ten minutes," as she walked out of the room.

The phone only rang twice before it was answered.

"Hello?" Becky said.

"Hey honey," I said, "it's me."

"How is my little Mondavi doing?" was her first, and probably only, question.

"Well...," I said reluctantly, with a crackle in my voice, "he is not doing so well babe."

I did not want to be the one giving her the bad news, I did not want to be in this situation. She already had so much to deal with, and I did not want her to worry about this too. But yet, here we were, and there was no other solution than to deal with it. Although I tried to be tough, I could not resist the tears that ran down my face as I started to explain to her what the veterinarian told me. The silence on the other side revealed her pain and sadness. Mondavi had been with her for seventeen years.

Although heartbreaking, I believed putting him down now was the most humane thing to do, and the veterinarian agreed, but ultimately it was Becky's decision. I was willing to do whatever she wanted me to do.

"Okay," she finally said after a long episode of silence.

"But bring him back home so we can bury him in the backyard next to Asti."

"Okay," was all I could get out.

Becky's words *'bring him back home'* were the straw that broke the camel's back, and tears freely streamed over my face. We both cried on the phone, not much was said. Although we were miles apart, during this moment of sadness it felt as if we were sitting right next to each other. Her head on my shoulder, my arms around her, together, supporting one another through this difficult time.

"I will be home as soon as I can," I promised her.

The veterinarian gave me the option to have him in my lap when she would give him the lethal injection, or to have it done in the back. She explained that she would first give him medicine to make him sleepy. Then, when he was asleep, she would administer the lethal injection that would ultimately stop his heart from beating.

"He will feel absolutely no pain at all," she promised me, "and I will be here with you all the time."

The last thing I could do for Mondavi was to be there for him when he would breathe his last breath, when he would move from this life to the next.

"Ok" I said, "I would like to be with him when he dies."

His white fur with little curls was still dirty in certain spots from the unfair battle he fought last night in that cold, wet field. His breathing was calm now. Shallow, but harmonious. His little broken body laid in my lap. My right hand was supporting his small head, his eyes were closed. My left hand was stroking along his body. There was a small area on his left front paw where they had shaved off some of his fur to insert the IV. The vet explained that they gave him some calming medication and fluids already,

"Just to make him feel a little better," she explained.

I continued to stroke his fur; long, gentle strokes from his neck down to his hind legs.

"I am giving him some medicine now that will make him sleepy," she said as she attached a syringe to the IV-port. She slowly pushed the plunger deeper into the syringe, injecting the medicine into his little body.

"We will wait about five minutes to make sure he is in a deep sleep," she explained as she detached the empty syringe from the IV-port.

I continued to run my fingers through his white curly fur. I knew the moment was getting closer for me to let him go. My hands started to shiver, and my vision was getting blurry from the excess liquid building up in the corners of my eyes. My heart pounding fast as I swallowed more frequently, trying to suppress my emotions.

"I am now giving him the medicine that will stop his heart from beating," she explained as she attached another syringe to his IV. This one had less fluid inside the chamber than the first one. She delicately pushed the ruthless poison inside his body. Soon it would take over and cause the irreversible death of our Mondavi.

"I will continue to listen to his heart," she said, as she placed her small stethoscope on his chest.

While I continued to caress him, I noticed his muscles relaxing. The weight of his tiny little body started to weigh heavier in my arms. My heart broke into a thousand little pieces. I knew he was gone and it felt like ravaging knives inside my chest. My tears fell silently onto his white fur.

"His heart has stopped beating," she delicately delivered the brutal message.

I did not call home, I did not call Becky, I could not find the courage to face the truth. Mondavi was in a box on the passenger seat. The veterinarian made a paw imprint in gypsum and wrote his name on the back. They were very kind, but their compassion did not make my pain easier or less difficult to deal with. My drive home was silent and long. While navigating through traffic, my soul cried for the loss of our little friend. My heart was heavy, as tears traced along my face. I could not help but to blame myself for this.

If I would have looked just a little longer outside, I might have found him.

I knew that Mondavi would go soon anyway, since he was so old, but I had hoped that Becky did not have to witness that. That she would not have to deal with the pain and the grief of losing him.

***

Becky, the boys, and I sat silently on the couch. We held hands, put our arms around each other and we cried. Mondavi's broken body was in a box on the table in front of us.

"I am taking him outside," I said as I stood up.

"Why don't you guys stay here with Mama, okay?"

"Okay," Connor and Dane responded.

Becky placed a kiss on the tips of her fingers. Slowly she moved her hand to the box and delicately rested it on top. Softly she whispered,

"Bye buddy, we will miss you".

My hand touched the side of her face. Becky looked up, her eyes red, soft tears rolling down her cheeks. I kissed her lips. No words were said, we all knew. Connor and Dane stared at the ground. I placed my hand on top of their heads followed by a soft kiss. With the box under my arm, I turned around and walked out.

I buried his body between the two large trees in our backyard, right next to Asti. I dug a hole earlier, right next to his gravesite, so they could rest next to each other. They had known each other for many years.

A little bump of dirt marked his grave.

The boys had gathered some wildflowers earlier, and I gently placed them on top of it.

Eighteen

Doctor Freeman's face showed intense signs of stress. The sparkle of joy I normally detected in his eyes was gone, or at least not noticeable. Although he smiled, anyone could see that it was fake. I knew that whatever he was going to tell us, was not going to be good news, maybe even devastating. He faced us, his back straight, and his hands in his lap. Becky and I, as always, were sitting next to each other holding hands. We were staring at him, waiting for the barrage of news.

Would it be the firing squad or just a stoning?

We had been going in and out the ER and interventional radiology more and more frequently lately.

"The restaging scan and MRI left me with some concerns," Doctor Freeman stated.

With our eyes locked on him, we sat still like statues.

"First the good news," he said.

"The MRI shows us that there is still no activity or growth of the leptomeningeal disease," as his smile appeared.

"Well, that's good, right?" Becky said.

"Yes, it is great news," Freeman confirmed. "The pulse dosing is working."

Becky looked at me and smiled.

"Although certain areas show improvement," Freeman continued, "there is more widespread activity throughout different organs."

He explained that they had found new tumors on her liver and in her right lung. Although the main tumor in her left lung had no growth, now there were new spots in her left and right lung, indicating progression of the disease. The cancer in her bones had also spread more along her spine.

"I think that the pulse dosing of Tarceva is doing a great job in attacking the leptomeningeal disease, but it allowed the cancer in other areas of the body to grow," he explained.

"I talked to Doctor Crawford and he recommended changing the Tarceva to 300 mg every other day."

We knew that he and Doctor Crawford were in frequent contact to discuss Becky's situation. It was good to know they both were open-minded about maintaining their communication.

"Roy, I also think that your research about the impact of adding Avastin to the treatment plan, is something we should try," he continued.

Our drive home was silent. Both of us stared silently through the windshield, our hands together with our fingers entangled. My thumb stroked the back of her hand delicately.

***

"The pain is really bad, sweetie!" Becky said.

Her eyes filled with tears and her lips pressed together as if she were trying to push down the increasing agony. Her hand rubbed her left shoulder, rocking forth and back in bed.

Over the last couple of days Becky's breathing started to become more difficult, and we were planning to go back to interventional radiology for another thoracentesis this week. This shoulder pain had started getting worse the day before. Becky and I both assumed that this was caused by a wrong move with her arm or something like that, but that morning, the pain rapidly became alarming. Besides the pain in her left shoulder, her left arm had swelled up to an unacceptable proportion; it was almost double in size. Becky was rocking back and forth to ease the pain. I determined it was time for action.

"I am going to take you to the ER sweetie," I said. "This is getting out of control."

"Maybe we should try some more painkillers to see if that helps before we go," Becky responded.

"Honey," as I turned around to face her directly, "besides the pain, look at your arm. It is swelling up like crazy."

The sad look in her eyes showed her agreement, but she just did not want to go. I sat down, right next to her, and placed my hand in hers.

"I know you don't want to go sweetie, but we really need to see what is going on."

"Okay," she reluctantly gave in.

The ER was starting to look like our second home. We spent too much time there. While the ER doctor completed his assessment, I stood back in the corner and observed. Since this ER doctor was unaware of Becky's situation, she had to explain almost everything from the beginning. Seeing Becky giving her own history, hearing her voice explaining what was going on, made me again realize what a horrible situation she was in. Less than a year ago, her life had been without many bumps, no sharp turns, and no dramatic situations. Suddenly, it all changed and now she was on this horrific journey from which no escape was possible. Becky was stronger and fought more fiercely than many ever could. Many would have collapsed under the pressure, but she was still standing, armed, ready for the continued battle in this unfair war.

The chest X-ray showed, once again, a large amount of fluid behind her lungs. Interventional radiology was contacted for another thoracentesis. I think by now it must have been the tenth or eleventh time in just a few months that they had to drain fluids from her lungs. After the thoracentesis, her shortness of breath was relieved. Shortly thereafter, an ultrasound was completed of her shoulder-neck area.

While we were waiting for the results in the ER-room, IV-medication was ordered for pain control. Over the last several weeks, it seemed that Becky's pain continued to get worse and more intense. The pain was all over her body in her neck, spine, bones, and chest. Becky didn't like the oral pain medications because they were knocking her out, but she seemed to tolerate the IV pain medication better.

I was sitting on one side of the bed with the railing down, my hand in hers. She was still in a lot of pain in her shoulder-neck area, but the IV medications seemed to take the edge off. The ER doc came back into the room, holding a paper in his hand.

"I have the ultrasound results here," he said, "and it seems you have a large blood clot in your left subclavian vein."

He moved closer to the bed and sat down on the edge of it.

"That explains the swelling and pain you have," he explained.

"It will be important to get you started on some blood-thinners and we will keep you here for observation."

Becky looked at me with sad eyes. I knew she did not want to stay another night here at the hospital.

"I also talked to Doctor Freeman," he said, "and he wants some restaging imaging done, and since we are keeping you here, I am going to schedule all that for tomorrow."

"Where did this blood clot come from?" Becky asked.

"Cancer patients are more prone to get those because of the disease process," he explained.

"It is a very common problem we see, but also easy to manage with medication."

Becky would get Enoxaparin injections twice a day. That would help dissolve the blood-clot and also prevent other clots from developing.

It seemed that more complications were starting to develop. It was depressing to see that, on one hand things were getting better, or at least they seemed to get better, but on the other hand, more complications popped up that caused all kinds of other issues. Now she had suddenly developed this blood clot in her neck.

We were waiting for the transfer from the ER to the floor. Sometimes this would take hours, depending on how busy they were on the floor and if the empty rooms were cleaned or not. Becky seemed to be resting comfortably, so I decided to go to the ER employee breakroom to check my mailbox since it had been a couple of weeks since I had worked.

The breakroom had a large rectangle table. At this table we had our roll call whenever there was a shift change. It was still covered with papers from earlier that evening. Food crumbs, napkins, and plastic silverware were scattered all over the table from the staff eating there. The smell of recently microwaved food lingered around the room.

Something Mexican, I thought, enjoying the aroma.

The mailboxes for all the nurses were on the left side of the room, right next to the entrance. Since they were alphabetized, my mailbox was in the middle towards the bottom. I retrieved a stack of papers, most of them single sheets. But an odd, thick smaller shape in the middle of the pile immediately grabbed my attention. I held the stack of papers by one corner between my thumb and index finger, letting it hang down over the table, and a smaller thick envelope fell out.

The front just said *'ROY'* and my name was underlined. The envelope was closed. On the back it said *'S.'* I pushed my index finger into the corner of the envelope and ripped it open. I retrieved a card from inside the envelope. It had a picture of a young boy, around 7 years old, wearing motorcycle goggles, a red cape, oversized red gloves, hands at his sides, standing tall and brave. The handwritten message on the inside touched me, very deeply:

You are a superhero.

I do not know how you do it.

I am so sorry about Becky, but you take care of her and your kids.

I know I would not be able to do this.

I think you have super-powers.

It is amazing to see how committed you are,

and how you take care of Becky and your boys.

– Stephanie

My walls that surrounded me, that protected me from all the attacks, all the negative assaults, crumbled down into a pile of rubble. Someone saw the pain I was enduring. Someone noticed the battles I fought in secret, especially out of sight from Becky and my boys. My soul cried so many times, broke, fell to pieces, and almost bled to death. But every time, before facing Becky or my boys, I would pick up those pieces, strengthen my walls, and appear as if nothing could tear me down. But in all reality, I broke many times, just without anyone noticing it. I cried alone, I screamed alone, I worried alone, I grieved alone. This unexpected note from one of my fellow nurses touched me in the soft spot. Although emotional, it brought me great joy that someone, totally unexpected, confirmed that I was doing the right thing.

Doctor Freeman was sitting down on the plastic chair on the opposite side of the bed, closest to the door. His back straight and his hands folded in front of him as if he were praying. I sat on the bed, right next to Becky. Both of us were focusing on what he was going to tell us since the MRI and CT-scan were completed earlier that morning. Normally he did his rounds in the morning, but I think he wanted to spend some extra time with us to explain what was going on.

The MRI revealed that the leptomeningeal disease was still no longer detectable. This was great news, but both Becky and I knew that there was more coming. The primary tumor in Becky's left upper lung seemed to be at a standstill, but there were many new smaller tumors. Several new spots were seen on the scan in her left lung, in her right lung, along the vertebrae of her spine, and other boney parts throughout her body. The tumor on her liver had almost doubled in size, and so had other tumors on her bones.

One battle was won, but five were lost. Doctor Freeman decided to go into a very long and detailed discussion about options. The only additional option left was chemotherapy, and he was not a fan of putting Becky through the horrific side-effects of chemo. He made clear that he was concerned that Becky's quality of life would diminish to almost nothing, and that the side-effects of chemo would probably kill her.

"I will do whatever you want to do," he told Becky, "but I think your quality of life will be horrible, and I want to prevent that."

He was silent for a moment, then continued to make his point.

"What good is it for any person to live a couple months longer if those months are filled with pain and agony?"

Becky and I both agreed with him that chemo would not be the solution.

***

It was nice to finally be out of that hospital room. We were driving back home with both windows down. Even though the cooler air gave us a chill now and then, the rush of fresh air caressing our skin was exhilarating. Becky's hand was holding mine, placed on the center console between us. The discharging oncologist agreed to send Becky home with a PCA pump so she could self-administer the IV pain medication. Hopefully now she would be able to control her pain better.

The last four days in the hospital had been brutal with too much negative news. I knew that the boys were also getting more concerned about what was going on. They noticed that we left the house more frequently to go to the hospital. They did not ask many questions, but I was concerned about them. Soon, I would have to spend some time with them and give them up to date about the situation and answer any questions they might have.

The evenings were still nice and cool at this time of the year. Soon summer would arrive with its sticky humidity and temperatures in the 100s that would make being outside miserable. The air would be so thick that it stuck to your skin like glue. Hot air, thick and heavy, made it hard to breath. At those times you could almost chew the air. That night it was nice outside, in the mid-60s. We were sitting outside on our porch, Becky was drinking a warm cup of green tea with local organic honey, I was sipping on a nice glass of red wine. The kind that would *'suck the moist from your tongue'*. Becky's favorite.

The boys were inside, playing a game on their X-box. It was in these moments where Becky and I would just sit together. She would lay her head on my shoulder and I would wrap my arm around her. Nothing was said, we just enjoyed being there together. I would rest my cheek on top of her head, and although her hair was gone, except for little stubbles, I could smell her scent. I closed my eyes and inhaled her fragrance. We communicated without words. Soul to soul, heart to heart. While we were sitting there, our bodies connected, our souls entangled, I tried to imagine, just for a moment, what it would feel like to be in her shoes.

Many times I prayed to God to spare her from this disaster. I asked Him many to give it to me instead. Becky did not deserve this. She was an amazing woman with a kind soul. If someone had to die, it should be me, not her. But it seemed that He had a different plan.

I remembered Lisa and Becky talking, many months ago, when Becky was just recently diagnosed with cancer. Lisa told Becky,

"I am so mad at God right now! Why is He doing this!"

Becky's response was amazing, and although she did understand Lisa's frustration, she said,

"God is not a bad person; it is not his fault."

It was the weekend, so the boys were able to stay up later. Becky had just gone to bed and the boys rushed into our bedroom for a goodnight kiss. After all the hugs and kisses they could collect, they ran back to the living room to continue their game. We had no clue about the game they were so pumped about. It had something to do with plants and zombies fighting each other. Becky seemed to do much better with her new PCA pump. She had not used it much yet, but whenever pain started to creep up on her, she would push the button for a quick release of medication that worked almost instantly.

I also had to give Becky her new medication, the blood-thinner shots, twice a day. This medication had to be injected in the abdominal area, just under the skin, not into a muscle or a vein. The needles were very small, like an insulin needle, and Becky always told me they did not really hurt.

After I cleaned her skin with an alcohol pad, I grabbed one of the prefilled syringes from the box, pinched some of Becky's skin between my index finger and thumb and removed the protective cap from the needle. Then, as I brought the needle closer to her skin, right before I would insert it, I said,

"Here's the poke."

I advanced the needle through her skin, about half an inch deep. Then slowly I pushed the medicine out of the syringe. She rolled on her side, I pulled her comforter over her shoulder, placed my hand on the side of her face, rubbed my thumb over her cheek, leaned forward and kissed her.

"I love you babe," I said, followed by another kiss.

"I love you too honey," she confirmed while her eyes made my heart melt.

"I am going to sit with the boys for a little, ok?" I told her.

"Okay honey," she said with a big smile.

She raised her hand and stroked the side of my face, her eyes bright filled with sweet love. I left our door open a crack, just enough for me to hear her if she needed me.

The boys were both sitting on the ottoman, right next to each other. Making movements with their whole bodies and their hands that were holding the game controllers. When their characters in their game turned left, turned right, jumped or had to crouch, so were Connor and Dane. It was a quite funny show to watch. I sat behind them in the large chair, wondering who came up with the idea for a game where zombies were fighting plants. About a half hour into the game observation, I told the boys to pause their game so we could talk for a moment.

Both controllers went down and the boys turned around on the ottoman to face me. These were always the moments I had difficulty with, telling our boys what was going on. Most of the time it was bad news, but it was my responsibility to keep them informed. I did not want to burden Becky with this problem, she had enough to worry about. I felt that not informing them about what was going on with their mama would just be wrong. It was uncomfortable, difficult, emotional, and I always wondered: how much do you say, and how do you say it?

"Well, as you know, we had to go back to the hospital," I started to explain, both their eyes glued onto me.

"There are some good things, and there are some bad things," I began, as I breathed deeply in and out.

"Remember Mama had that cancer tumor in her neck that was really bad?" I asked.

Both Connor and Dane, eyes locked, not saying anything, just nodded.

"Well, it seems that that one is gone. They can't find it anymore."

The worry on their faces faded as their smiles appeared.

"And all the pain that Mama had in her neck and shoulder, turned out to be a large blood clot in her neck," I continued.

"What is a blood clot?" was Connor's immediate response.

Followed by Dane's question, "How do you get that out?"

After I explained how blood clots were formed and how we treat them, they both seemed relieved that it was an easy fix.

"But some of the scans they did when Mama was in the hospital showed some concerning developments," I forced myself to tell them.

"There are areas showing more activity, and overall they are worried, and it seems that the cancer is slowly spreading."

My stomach turned as I had to inform them about this. It broke my heart to tell them that the cancer was slowly growing. Connor and Dane understood all too well what was going on. Their eyes sad, their smiles turned into small lips.

"We have decided to continue with the treatment we are doing now and see what happens over the next several months," I explained.

Both of them stood up, Connor sat on my right knee, Dane on the left. Their arms were around my neck and my chest, my arms were around them. I kissed their little heads one at a time. Soft tears fell, we all felt horrible. I wished I could protect my boys from this painful journey, but we could not change the path we were on. We just sat there for a while, holding each other.

"You have to come to me and ask me any questions you have, okay?" I whispered.

Both their heads nodded on my shoulder.

Becky was all pumped up. I did not know where she got the energy from, but she found a ton of it somewhere. Today was my birthday and she had been organizing a party for the last couple of weeks. Her energy levels had been getting better ever since she received that PCA pump for pain control. Even Doctor Freeman had made a comment about it during one of the last visits. I knew Becky was on the phone with a lot of people trying to get things organized; she wanted to do something special for my birthday.

Around 4pm people started to come over. Everything was a big surprise to me. I was not planning on having a big birthday party, but Becky had different plans. She wanted to do this. I had not seen this amount of motivation in her for months. It was great to see her surrounded by all those who dearly loved her.

I remember that at one point one of her friends gave me a birthday present. A card was attached to it and, as I opened the card, Becky's friend made clear I should also open the present since it went well with the card. She also wanted me to read the card out loud. I ripped the paper off of the present, and I was holding my gift in my hands; superman underwear with a big 'S' on the front, bright blue with red lining. The card that came with the present was in the same style. A picture of superman flying through the air was on the front of it. Before I decided to read the card in theatrical style, I placed the underwear on top of my jeans where it would normally be worn, then, with the card in my right hand, I used my left hand to emphasize the theatrical performance.

I read the card: "On this glorious day…" in my best British accent, trying to outdo Hamlet, I started my performance. I do not remember what that card said exactly anymore, but the gist of it was that she thought I was superman for all the things I was doing for Becky and the boys. This was a very meaningful card, but the way I was performing, speaking with a British accent, Hamlet style, had everyone cracking up laughing. When I peeked to my right, where Becky was sitting, I saw tears rolling down her cheeks from laughter. Those tears were my best birthday present ever; seeing my girl laughing so hard that she was crying.

Becky had a special present for me. She handed me a box, wrapped in Christmas paper.

"Sorry honey," she said, "I couldn't find the birthday paper. I think we are out of it."

"No worries babe," I said as I gave her a quick kiss.

Slowly I started to unwrap the paper. A big brown box, taped shut with masking tape, revealed my next challenge. I opened the top of the box and as I peeked inside, I could see what it was. I smiled, choking, swallowing down my emotions. I turned my head, Becky's eyes glittering bright, filled with tears, her hand covering her mouth, covering her beautiful smile.

"Do you remember?" she asked with a broken voice, tears now rolling down her cheeks.

"Oh, yes, honey, I do," was all I could get out before I broke down.

Her head fell onto my shoulder, my head onto hers. Our arms held one another as our shoulders shivered and soft sobbing tears flowed. Total silence around us, no one spoke a word.

"Remember how I used to watch you play for hours?" she whispered.

"Yes, those were fun times," I said.

Back in 1998, when Becky and I just met, I moved to her townhouse. I had an old Nintendo game system, and I used to play a game called Zelda. Becky would sit on the couch behind me, watching me play the game and giving me all the instructions on where to go, what to do, what not to do, who to kill, and so forth. I was just moving the little guy in the game to wherever she wanted me to go. We spent hours playing this game together, but whenever I asked her if she wanted to play herself, she always responded,

"I don't know how to play that game. You do a much better job at it."

She would not touch the controller, but she loved to play together. That old Nintendo broke down a long time ago and we never replaced it. When the boys were old enough, we bought them an Xbox.

For this birthday, Becky went out of her way to find an old Nintendo with all the old games, especially Zelda games. Although that was the physical present in the box, it represented a much more valuable gift of memories.

Nineteen

Slowly I rolled up my eyelids. It was still dark outside. I reached over to my phone on the nightstand. The time was 2:31am.

Why am I waking up?

Still confused, I turned onto my right side to curl up with Becky. My hand reached over and landed down on the comforter, all the way down to the mattress. Another pat, now further away, nothing. Patting up, patting down, nothing. I sat up, looked around and no one was there.

"What the…" I whispered under my breath.

I jumped out of bed to see where she was.

Maybe the bathroom?

As I walked through the hallway, I found the bathroom empty. I made my way to the kitchen, no one there. The living room was completely dark, so I couldn't see anything. I turned on the standing lamp that was placed in the corner of the room. As the illumination spread through the area, I saw her sitting on our chair in her multi-colored robe, legs tucked underneath her, awake as can be, silently, just smiling and staring at me.

"Honey, what are you doing?" I asked, still sleepy.

"Nothing," she answered with a bright voice.

"Why are you sitting here?" I asked her, still confused.

"Just because," she replied nonchalantly.

She sounded confused and out of the norm. Something was not right. I sat down next to her and placed my hand in hers. She just smiled as she wrapped her fingers around my hand and got a firm hold of it.

"Let's go to bed babe," I said.

"Okay," she replied. She stood up and pulled my hand.

"Let's go," she said.

We walked back to our bedroom. As she laid down on her right side, I crawled behind her and placed my arm around her. We kissed goodnight as if nothing had happened.

During the next few days there were more of these awkward episodes where I could not find her. She would be sitting outside, in the basement, in the bathroom, or in my office. She acted more confused by the day. My fear increased at night when I was asleep. I was worried that she would get back up again, and although I normally would wake up, I was scared she would be so quiet that I did not hear her.

I remember that the radiology-oncologist explained that the brain radiation would cause some confusion, but I did not like this situation. I asked some of our family members and our friend Lisa if they could help out and sleep over at our house, just to have another adult there in case something happened.

The home-health nurse already asked me several times to change Becky's care from home-health to home-hospice. They would be able to stop by more often and stay as long as we needed.

"I know Doctor Freeman will approve it," she said.

Although I hated the word 'hospice'...to me it means the final step...I thought it would be helpful to have a little more assistance and agreed with the home-health nurse to change her status.

***

BANG … BANG … BANG. What is that sound?
BANG … BANG … BANG. There it was again.

It sounded like someone was banging something on our windows, but the boys were both sitting in front of me, on the ottoman, playing a game on the X-box. They both had their headsets on, so they didn't hear anything. Becky was trying to get some sleep since she was up most of the morning. We had all eaten some lunch in our bedroom, while sitting on our bed. Everyone had a plate in their lap, surrounding Becky, so we could eat together. Becky and I always made it a habit to eat together as a family at the dining room table. It allowed for quality family time where we could talk about our day and anything else under the sun.

"Research has shown that eating dinner at the dining room table as a family, creates socially strong people," Becky would always preach.

Although I was not sure about the *'research'* part, I agreed with her about having that family time at the table. So, we always tried to at least have dinner together. Ever since Becky was more bedridden, we barely had sit-down dinners at the table, so we decided to just sit down with her in our bedroom.

BANG … BANG … BANG. There it was again.

I stood up, turned my head to the left, then to the right, to hear better and determine where the noise was coming from. I tapped Connor on his shoulder as I stood up. He turned his head and looked at me. Without a sound I tapped my index finger vertically on my lips, indicating that they had to be silent. Connor paused their game. As the screen froze, Dane looked at him with big questioning eyes. Dane took off his headset and as he was ready to ask Connor what was going on, Connor pointed at me.

"What's going on Papa?" Dane asked.

"I hear a loud banging sound," I said, "but I am not sure where it is coming from."

I told the boys to keep their headsets off and stop the game for a moment. I started to investigate. With cat-like moves I glided through the living room toward the back of the house. Like a Ninja, I silently floated over the hardwood floor, turning and tilting my head to different directions, trying to pick up any turbulence in the air that could reveal the location of the disturbance. My main concern was Becky. I did not want anything or anyone waking her up. I froze at the top of the stairs. From there I could hear in almost every direction, and since the front door was only a few steps away, if the sound was coming from outside the house, I could get there fast.

Connor and Dane sat frozen on the ottoman, waiting for me to figure something out. Of course, nothing happened, so I continued my silent advance into the hallway, past the bathroom, the boys' rooms and towards our bedroom. I peeked into our bedroom from the hall, and I could see our bed. A shock bolted through my body, and I froze instantly, my head jerked back, my eyes squeezed to sharpen my sight. My eyebrows frowned. Our bed...empty.

Confused, I moved slowly forward into our bedroom. My mind was racing in high gear trying to figure out where Becky went. Before I could answer that question,

BANG ... BANG ... It was coming from our bedroom.

The sound was loud and clear, and it was coming from our windows. I was confused, scared, and nervous, with adrenaline rushing through my veins to prepare myself for God only knows what. My heart was thumping in my chest, my hands were shaking, and all my senses were on full alert.

I stepped into our bedroom and stood next to an empty mattress. The comforter was pushed to the side, and the wrinkles of the fitted sheet provided evidence that it was recently used. My eyes focused forward, aimed at the windows. There she was, standing there, facing the window. Her left hand rested against the wooden window frame, her right hand held her PCA-pump. She was standing motionless, silently staring out the window. She did not hear me come in and was not aware I was standing behind her.

I was still wondering what was going on.

Why was she out of our bed? Why was she standing there? What was that noise?

I started to step towards her, and right before I was going to ask her what she was doing, she raised her right hand, holding the PCA-pump, her fingers clamped around its edges. Her knuckles white and the increased definition of the tendons of her hand proved that she was squeezing it hard, holding it as tight as possible. With her left hand still holding on to the frame, she started to slowly bring back her right hand, overhead, and then, full force forward …

BANG … BANG … BANG.

She slammed the PCA pump on the glass of the window trying to break it.

"Honey," I said calmly, trying not to scare her,

"what are you doing?" I was confused, rattled by her actions.

She slowly turned around, her right arm still in the air, ready for another attack at the window. Her sweet face showed pain. The light in her eyes was dim, she was confused, her smile was lost.

"I need to get out of here," she declared.

Her voice was frantic and filled with fear.

"I need to get out of this place, now!" as she turned around for another attack on the window.

"Babe, stop," I said, calm but concerned.

She was only a couple of steps away from me, so I reached her within seconds. Gently I placed my hand around her lower arm to bring it down from the attack position. I leaned my body against her, kissed her cheek while my left hand reached around her waist, and placed my arm around her. She did not resist my actions, and she seemed to calm down.

"I have to get out of here," she said, her eyes desperate and on a mission.

"I need to get to a hospital so they can cure me!" her hands shook, her eyes screamed for help.

My heart was heavy. She was so desperate, her pain so deep. My soul cried on the inside, my eyes filled with tears, but I had to stay strong. I had to stay clear and calm. She was very confused. I had never seen her like this, so aggressive, and with so much desperation in her eyes. I needed to calm her down. I walked back to the bed with her and she sat down on the edge with me, but she did not give up.

"We really need to leave here as soon as possible," she continued, making movements again to get back up.

Her confused state of mind and her determination gave her unexpected strength. I had a hard time holding on to her. I knew I should not try to wrestle her because that would make the situation worse. It was obvious she was very confused. Maybe it was the radiation, maybe it was the cancer that was growing, maybe it was the medicine, or maybe it was all those factors combined.

While I tried to calm her, my brain was searching for solutions. I knew that Ativan would calm her, but that was in the fridge in the kitchen. I had to get over there, draw it up in a syringe, get back and give it to her through her port. But if I left her alone, God only knew what she would do, but I had no other solution.

"Honey, you stay right here, okay," I said,

"I have to get something and I will be right back," as I placed my hand on her cheek and kissed her lips.

"Okay," she said.

As fast as I could, I walked towards the kitchen, but when I opened the fridge, I could hear it again,

BANG ... BANG ... BANG.

I grabbed the vial of Ativan from the fridge, a needle, a syringe, and a handful of alcohol wipes.

I will have to do it in our room.

I started to rush back towards our bedroom, when suddenly the front door opened; it was the home-health nurse.

"Oh my God," I exclaimed, "am I happy to see you!"

"What's going on?" she asked.

"Becky is very confused," I said. "She is very..."

BANG ... BANG ... BANG ...

"What is that noise?" the nurse asked.

"Becky is banging on the windows trying to break the glass. She keeps yelling that we have to leave and get to the hospital," I explained rapidly.

"You go draw up that Ativan, I will go and calm down Becky," she said as she dropped her bag onto the floor and came up the stairs.

As I started to draw up the Ativan, I could hear them talking, but could not understand the words. With the syringe in my right hand, needle exposed and aiming up, I picked up the vial and as I brought it closer to the syringe, I noticed my hands shaking. I needed to calm down, so I closed my eyes and tried to clear my thoughts. I took a couple of deep breaths in and then slowly out, focusing my energy on this moment, this task. I drew up a dose of Ativan and placed the vial back in the fridge. I grabbed a saline flush and walked back to our bedroom.

The nurse had Becky calmed down. She was sitting on the edge of the bed again. Her right hand was still clinging on to the PCA pump, her knuckles still white. She kept saying that she had to leave and that they would have a cure for her at the hospital. Then Becky started to plead with me. God, it made me feel horrible.

"But honey, I know that if we leave, they can get me healthy in the hospital," she said.

At that moment, I remembered when my dad had bypass surgery and they had used Demerol for pain-control, but he reacted wrong to it and started having hallucinations. I remembered visiting him at the hospital and he said,

"Those damn Germans stole my veins."

My dad used to be in the navy, and he thought he was on a warship and that the German doctors stole his veins and replaced them with plastic tubes. He had suction tubes coming from his chest, but he was convinced those were placed by German surgeons after they stole his veins. The cardiologist told me not to argue with him, but to just ignore it, or go along with it. As soon as they stopped the Demerol, his hallucinations disappeared. I planned to have the same approach with Becky's current situation; I would not argue with her.

"I know honey," I said while I started to administer the Ativan.

As soon as the Ativan got into her system, she started to relax and laid back down in our bed.

To see my sweetheart this confused, so desperate in her mission to get out of this situation, broke my heart. The feeling of complete loss of control made me feel helpless and alone. The brutal realization that this cancer had taken over my girl, was devastating and horrifying, but regardless, I was still trying to be her rock. Still trying to be her light in this dark scary night.

The home-health nurse and I stood in the kitchen while Becky was resting in our bedroom. She placed her hand on my forearm and with a concerned look in her eyes, she said,

"Listen Roy, I really think it is time to take her to hospice."

My heart stopped. I always said that I would take care of Becky in our home until the end. Taking her to hospice was something I never wanted to do; it felt like I was giving up.

"Look," she continued, "look what happened this afternoon," she paused.

Then she raised her index finger to make sure I understood the importance of the next sentence.

"If I would not have come into the house this afternoon, God knows what could have happened," her eyes now strict but concerned.

"Becky could have broken that glass and cut herself, or worse..." and she stopped right there.

Deep inside I knew she was right, I could not do it by myself any longer, but I had the feeling I was failing her. I promised her that I would take care of her. I promised her that I would get her better. She had asked me not to let her die. How could I promise all that and now fail my mission to take care of my sweetheart? My soul was screaming, my heart was being ripped to pieces, the inside of my chest felt like someone was slicing it with a sharp knife. Tears started to roll down my face. The nurse placed her hand on my shoulder, and with one short sentence she convinced me.

"It is time for you to be Becky's husband again, and stop being her nurse."

Oh my God this was so hard, so difficult. I did not want to let her go. I knew hospice was the end. I did not want it to be the end. I wanted her here with me and my boys, not in some distant strange building far from home. I want to hold her every night and kiss her goodnight. I wanted to travel with her to the places we said we would go. I did not want her to go. I did not want her to die. Why not me? Why her? Let me die, not her.

Why…why …

The nurse placed her arms around me as a sea of tears flooded down my cheeks, my shoulders shivering with every breath. My soul wept for it knew it was going to lose its mate. It was the most difficult decision to make, but I knew it was the right one. I called Lisa to see if she could stay with Connor and Dane. The phone rang only a few times before she answered.

"What's up."

"Well," as I started to talk, my lips began to shake, swallowing down my tears, my voice broken.

"Lisa, I am going to take Becky to hospice…"

The silence on the phone was brutally painful. Lisa was there from the beginning. She was utterly well aware of the downhill slope we were on. She knew what it meant to go to hospice.

"Can you come over and take care of the boys?" I asked.

"I am on my way," she said with a cracked voice.

I hung up and browsed through my contacts to find the dispatch number for the hospital ambulance. Larry answered the phone. Over the years I worked there, we became close. I took a deep breath in and cleared my throat and tried to sound as normal as I could.

"Larry, it's Roy…" I said.

"It is Becky, I need to take her to hospice. Can you send a crew without lights and siren please?"

"Absolutely, I will dispatch them right now," he said.

"And Roy, if you ever just need to talk, you know where you can find me, ok?"

"Ok, thanks Larry," I responded.

I wiped my tears, trying to compose myself again. There were still two difficult tasks at hand. First, I had to tell the boys. Then I had to tell Becky. Connor and Dane were sitting on the ottoman. Their little eyes filled with questions and worries. They observed and watched the last several hours unfold in front of them. Their mama was acting differently, the home-health care nurse was calling people, Papa was crying and upset, now Lisa was on her way. They must have been well aware that something was going to happen, they were just unsure about what it was. As I walked into the living room, their little eyes were glued onto me, waiting for information and clarification. I sat down, both Connor and Dane hanging on my lips.

I explained that Mama was going to a different hospital. They understood this news was far from normal. There was too much commotion in the house, too many people, too many phone calls. The house was saturated with awkwardness, but they knew that I would always tell them everything and that I would never keep anything from them.

"Lisa will be here to take care of you guys, okay?" I explained.

They both nodded.

"I am not sure when I will be back. I might stay the night with mama, but for sure. I will call you tonight if I am not coming home," I told them.

They both stood up and gave me a big hug. I kissed both their cheeks.

"I love you guys."

"Love you too, Papa" they both said.

The ambulance arrived as requested, without lights and siren. Before they could knock on the door, I stepped outside to welcome them. I knew both medics well, as we had worked together for many years. They walked up to me, and one by one they hugged me. No words were said, no words were needed. We all knew the situation. We all knew where we were going. I asked them not to use the word hospice, but facility. Becky was already confused as it was, there was no need to make her anymore disoriented. Since the hallway to our bedroom was very narrow, they placed the gurney in the living room. I was going to carry Becky to the gurney from our bedroom.

I could hear Becky and the home-health nurse talking as I progressed through the hallway. I did not like this, I did not want to do this. I forced myself forward and stepped into the bedroom. The home-health nurse was sitting on the bed, next to Becky, facing her. Becky's head turned around towards me the moment I stepped into the room. Her eyes bright, her lips smiling.

"Hey sweetie," she joyfully said.

It seemed that the confusion had subsided for a moment.

"Hey Babe," I responded.

"The medics are here to take you to a special hospital, okay?"

My heart was beating in my chest as the words left my lips and fear creeped under my skin. I was afraid of how she might react.

"Okay honey," she said.

Relieved that there was no argument, I leaned towards her. I kissed her lips. Her eyes were beautiful, no longer puzzled.

"I am going to carry you over there since they can't get the cot through the hallway."

She raised her arms in the air towards me, ready to be carried away. While I placed my right arm underneath her legs, and my left around her torso, she folded her arms around my neck and as I raised her with ease from the bed, she kissed me on the cheek.

"I love you crazy Dutchman," she said.

As she pulled her body closer to mine, I strengthened my grip to hold her tight. Our souls close together, our bodily warmth intermingled. I closed my eyes as I started to feel the tears pushing through, I swallowed down the heavy lump in my throat.

The medics started to place security straps around Becky's body, as they explained step by step to her what they were doing.

"Just putting some seatbelts on you for safety," as the medic clicked the strap around her hips.

Everything went well until they rolled the cot outside, towards the ambulance.

"Honey," Becky said,

"let's just stay home sweetie, I don't wanna go to the hospital anymore."

I could feel her squeezing my hand. Oh my God, that tore my heart into pieces. I wanted to give in and keep her home, but I knew that her confusion was too much for me to handle by myself. Even though I really wanted to keep her home, I knew this was the best solution for now.

"I know honey," I said, "let's just check it out and if you don't like it, we can just come right back, okay?" I tried to calm the situation.

"Okay," she responded with a smile.

The cot was locked in place, I was sitting right next to her, holding her hand, and one of the medics was sitting at her head. He started to get her blood-pressure, listened to her lungs and got all the other vital signs that were needed to complete the paperwork. I could hear the medic up front call in the report to dispatch.

"We are in route with the spouse of an employee, stage IV lung cancer, confusion, currently cooperative..."

It sure is different when you are sitting in the back of an ambulance and you are not working.

It was late afternoon and the sun was ready to settle for the night. We were at the end of the summer and cooler days had arrived again. The ambulance turned into the parking lot. I recognized the hospice house as I had been here many times as a paramedic. It was a white ranch-style building. The main entrance faced the street, with a wide and long overhang and brick columns placed on both sides. We were on the south-side of the building, at the ambulance entrance. As we came in through the side door, the hospice nurse welcomed us. She leaned over to Becky, placed her hand on hers, and with a gentle and kind voice said,

"You must be Becky."

Becky looked up, smiled, but said nothing. I walked these hallways many times as a medic, handing over the care of a patient to one of the hospice nurses. All those times I was not expecting to ever be here myself or for any of my loved ones, yet here we were. We were walking the corridors that led to the point of no return. Before I left our home, I called the family to inform them. Some of them got her before we did and were already sitting by the room that was assigned to Becky.

As the hospice nurses started to get Becky ready in her room, they asked me to come to the front office to complete some paperwork.

"I will be right back babe, okay?" I told Becky.

"I just have to fill out some paperwork."

Becky's eyes filled with fear, she was scared. Like a little girl that goes to the doctor but doesn't want to be there. Scared for a shot or whatever they might do. Becky had the same fear in her eyes. I tried to calm her, placed my hand on her right cheek, kissed her, and said,

"It will only take a minute, okay sweetie? I will be back before you know it."

"Ok," she hesitated.

After I was done with all the official forms and paperwork, I went back to Becky's room. She was sitting upright in her bed, surrounded by family members. Her eyes were glazed over, she was non-responsive. The nurse explained that they had to give her some Haldol since she was becoming increasingly confused and combative after I left the room. I sat down at her feet, placed my hand on her left lower leg, and said,

"Hey Sweetie."

She looked at me with the deer in the headlight look, non-responsive, blank, empty. The Haldol was in full effect. It was horrible to see her like that.

During my meeting in the front office, besides going over all the legal issues and insurance, we had a discussion about the prognosis in regard to Becky's stay at hospice. They explained that all medication would be stopped, except for those that actually caused comfort and decreased the pain.

"Our main goal is to have her without any pain and as comfortable as humanly possible," she stated.

The only medicine they would continue at this time was the PCA-pump with pain medicine, and the steroids since these were decreasing the swelling in her brain.

"At a certain point in time during the next several days," the nurse continued, "Becky will have her *last supper,* as we call it."

The confusion in my eyes caused her to elaborate.

She explained that this *'last supper'* is a common phenomenon with terminally ill patients. Most patients that are close to dying will fall asleep after they stated that they had a good tasting dinner, and then they would not wake up anymore.

"This means that she will eat something and she will state that is the best thing she ever ate, and she would like more of it," the nurse explained.

"No matter what it is, she will love it. After that meal she will fall asleep and will not wake up."

"So, you mean that she will...be gone?" I asked.

"Yes, that is why we call it the *last supper*," she responded with a soft voice.

I raised my hand towards my face, placed it over my mouth and sighed.

Twenty

It had been several hours since we arrived at Mercy Hospice. The effects of Haldol had worn off and Becky was more talkative. I was sitting in the recliner right next to her bed and as always, we were holding hands. Becky was talking with one of her siblings that was sitting on the little loveseat to her right, underneath the large window that had a view of the green grass field outside. The nurse was getting some vital signs and as she was getting ready to leave, she turned towards Becky and asked her what she wanted for dinner. After the choices were discussed, Becky let her know her decision. The nurse promised her that she would bring her food shortly.

"Is there anything else that you would like Becky?" she asked.

Becky almost jumped up in bed, she sat straight up, swung her arms into the air, wide open with palms up, big smile and a glitter of menace in her eyes.

"Well," she said, "I really would like to spend some nights alone with my husband."

Everyone in the room cracked up and started to laugh out loud. I just smiled when she looked at me.

"You can get all the alone time you need with your husband, sweetheart," the nurse responded.

In that moment, that was just funny for most, I realized the true meaning of that statement. Too many times, while Becky was in the hospital, I decided to stay with the boys. Her declaration to me was clear, I made up my mind. I would sleep here, with her, every night.

Most people might have thought that it was a funny statement, but Becky made it clear that she wanted some alone time with me. She was sick and tired of the sisters and the friends staying with her at nighttime. She wanted to hold my hand, kiss my lips before she would rest her soul, and she desired to wake up in the morning and see me next to her. At that moment she was probably even aware that her days were short and that she wanted to spend her last days with her husband, her soulmate, her love.

Becky had eaten her dinner and was asleep. It had been a stressful day and it was late. Most of the family had been there all day and were tired and ready to go home. We all walked to the main entrance. We hugged, kissed, and said goodbye. At that moment, that first day at hospice, we were one family again. We were all scared, we were all afraid for the future, but we were there to support each other, not to argue or blame others.

The hallway was empty and still as I walked back to Becky's room. The nurse's station was unmanned as they were probably with another patient. On both sides of the oversized hallway, were loveseats with coffee tables. Magazines were placed on each table. The appearance of this facility was very clean, serene with light colors on the walls, floors and furniture.

I had left Becky's door open a crack. I gently pushed it open, the soft light from the hallway snuck into the room, throwing long shadows over the floor onto the bed. At that moment, I stood there, staring at my wife, sleeping in a hospice bed, I realized she was never going to leave this room; she would die here.

The recliner was already perfectly positioned right next to her bed. The nurse had placed some sheets, blankets, and a couple of pillows on it. After I made my resting place for the night, I laid my body down. On my side first, placing my hand under my head, I just stared at Becky for a moment. As she laid there, calm and peaceful, I knew that her magnificent soul was harbored in this broken, sick, close-to-death body. Her sheer beauty manifested itself through her radiant presence, not through her physical appearance.

No words were needed, no sight required, just the pure sensation of her loving presence next to mine. A slow tear traveled calmly down my cheek. We talked for a while. Well, I was doing all the talking, and she was doing all the listening. I turned over onto my back, my hand in hers. I could hear her breathe, deep and slow. Our physical bodies might be separated by a wooden armrest and a metal side rail, but our souls were laying right next to one another, holding each other tight.

***

I opened the door and stepped into the building with resistance. It felt as if I were being pushed in. I did not want to be here. The hardwood floor was dark brown and recently cleaned or maybe oiled, since the scent of orange was still strong. A framed display with names, dates, and times was the first thing that caught my eye. Behind it, four chairs surrounded a small table on top of a rug. A box of tissues sat in the middle. To the right, there were white, French doors, probably leading to some offices. Straight ahead were stairs with green carpet leading to the second floor. To the left, an American flag, and a white high-top table with comfortable looking square chairs placed against the wall. Through the open doors I could see rows of pews.

My appointment was for 10 AM. That gave me time to take a shower, get the boys to school, and drive over here for this dreadful meeting. I stood there like a lost young boy that was abandoned by his parents in the middle of the mall. Within seconds a young lady emerged from the hallway to my right, from behind the French doors. She must have been warned by the chime that was activated when I opened the front door. She was professionally dressed in a women's pencil skirt suit, black heels, and white shirt. She smiled as she reached out her hand to shake mine.

"You must be Roy Slo, ehh, Slooth, ...?" as she started to try to pronounce my last name.

"Yes, I am," as I interrupted her attempt.

"Don't worry about it, not many get it right," I smiled, shaking her hand.

Yesterday the hospice nurse made it very clear that I needed to make arrangements soon. One of the first things I had to do was to make an appointment with a funeral home. Here I was, 10 AM, shaking the hand of someone that worked there. Not in my wildest dreams did I expect to be in this situation at this time in my life. She was very kind and gentle with her words. We went straight ahead, up the stairs, and we sat down at a large round table in a spacious meeting room.

"Coffee?" she asked.

"Yes, please," I responded.

She placed the cup filled with liquid caffeine in front of me and sat down. In the middle of the table stood a rectangle sugar packet caddy, filled with packages of sugar and different sweeteners. I supplied my coffee with two Splenda's when she asked,

"One of the first things we need to discuss is if Becky is going to be buried or cremated?"

That question was a dagger straight into the heart. I really did not want to talk about this, but I had to be realistic. I closed my eyes for a second, deep breath in, slowly out.

I can do this.

Even though Becky and I never talked about this matter, never discussed any of these details, we knew what we wanted. I knew what she wanted, and she knew what I wanted when it would come to this.

"Becky is a free spirit," I said, "I am not going to put her in a box in the ground."

"Okay," she answered.

"She is going to the ocean," I continued, "right next to Grandma Freddie, swimming with the fishes."

She smiled. "Well, let's go look around," she said.

I just tried to keep my posture, tried not to break down. I kept telling myself I could do this. As I followed her through the rows of different caskets, I was shocked that there were so many choices. She stopped at some here and there, but none of them were suitable or worthy for my Becky and I turned them all down. Then she stopped and said,

"This one is frequently used when a younger person passes," she explained.

"As you can see, there is no finish on this light natural wood."

"Okay," I said, wondering about the uniqueness of it.

"This one comes with a big box of colored markers so everyone can leave a message on the casket," she explained.

"That's the one," I replied. "Unique, like Becky, perfect for the boys."

I opened the large front door, and as I was holding it open with my stretched arm, both Connor and Dane burst through the opening. Right next to the entrance was a small office. It was used by multiple people for different purposes. The door to that office was wide open, and as we walked by, the lady that was sitting behind the desk, stood up. I think she was a counselor of some sort, but the boys and I moved on, past the office, towards Becky's room.

"Hey guys," she said, trying to get their attention.

Connor and Dane stopped in the middle of their tracks. She gestured for them to come into the office. After I walked in and shook her hand, both boys felt comfortable enough to come in too. All she wanted to do, was to introduce herself to us and let us know she would always be available to talk. We sat down at the small table in the corner that was surrounded by a loveseat and two smaller chairs. She asked them if they wanted to talk to her or if they had any questions. Both boys looked at each other, shook their heads, and raised their shoulders. Connor responded for the both of them.

"If we have any questions, we ask Papa," he said. "We talk all the time."

Knowing that my boys trusted me in their quest for information or when they needed answers, proved to me that I had been doing the right thing by talking to them about everything that was going on with Becky.

We left her office and walked through the hallways to see Mama. Connor was on the left holding my hand, and Dane on the right holding my other hand. Although it is difficult as a parent to be open and honest to your kids in these situations, it is absolutely the right thing to do.

I was trapped between a rock and a hard place. On one hand I wanted to protect them from harm, both physically and mentally, but not giving the information about what is going on might be done to protect a child, but in the long run, you will cause more hurt, because they will figure it out. Then, when they have the feeling that you have been lying to them, you have a whole other problem on your hands. Telling them the truth and keeping them informed is hard, but it strengthens the overall relationship with your kids.

Connor, Dane and I walked through that hallway as one unit, as one team.

Becky was sitting upright in bed. Her eyes lit up the room the moment we walked in. She snuggled with the boys as they jumped on her bed. She reached one of her arms out towards me, and while the boys surrounded her body, she waved her fingers, telling me to come closer. She pulled me in as soon as I placed my hand in hers. She placed her other hand on the side of my face, kissed my lips, and said,

"Hey babe, I love you."

"Hey sugar, how are you?" I asked as I sat down in the same recliner next to her that was my bed earlier.

The boys were all over her and she loved every minute of it. They went on and on about what happened at school that day. Afterall, it was their first school day of the new year. It was always such a delight to see Becky's spirit lifted when her boys would appear.

There were three knocks on the door behind me, followed by a female voice,

"Knock, knock! Anyone home?"

Becky's eyes jumped wide open, since she recognized that voice.

"Oh my God, Angie!" she exclaimed.

"Look guys, it is Angie!"

Over the last year, Angie had been there with us, during the ups and downs, the smiles and the tears, the little joys, and mountains of pain. She was there not only to support Becky, but to support us as a unit. It was a joy to see her. Her positive spirit always put a smile on our faces. Even though she had many of her own problems, she always managed to make us feel better.

"I normally don't do this," she said, "visiting patients, but I just live around the corner from here, so…"

She stepped closer to the bed, then sat down at Becky's feet on the mattress.

"So, who is Connor, and who is Dane?" she asked as she clapped her hands softly together.

"I have heard everything about you!"

It was obvious she was a mom herself; she was great with kids.

In the 30-minute visit, her presence was worth so much more than the words she spoke. She cared and she was concerned. That was why she was there.

I walked her out to the front door. Both Connor and Dane gave her a big squeezing sandwich hug. They knew she was a good person. Becky folded her arms around her neck, and I could hear her whisper,

"Thank you for coming."

Angie and I walked through the hall and when she knew we were far enough away, she placed her hand on my shoulder and asked,

"Are you ok?"

It is amazing to realize that a simple touch can cause a cascade of reactions. It was not just the words that released the avalanche of emotions, it was the gentle touch. With that delicate contact, she told me that she understood how difficult this was, she understood the hardship, she understood the pain. I had to swallow down a lump before I could answer, and with a broken voice I declared the truth,

"This sucks."

The morning came too soon. The nights were too short caused by discomfort and frequent waking episodes. I tried to adjust my body that had been abused on this device of torture that was never designed for something known as a good night's sleep. Naps, yes, but nothing more than that. Becky had a restless night with many episodes of waking. Several times because of pain, but a quick push on the PCA button managed that. A couple of times she had to go to the bathroom and that was quite an undertaking since she barely could walk. So, we decided to have a bedside commode for her.

I opened my eyes and I could feel that burning sensation you feel when you have been crying for hours. I glanced over to my right, my arm was stuck between the recliner's armrest and Becky's bed. My hand was still resting on top of her hip. Her breathing was shallow, but regular. The rhythmic motion of her chest provided an unusual comfort.

Gently, I pulled my arm from between its trap. Due to the lack of blood-supply, my hand was completely numb. I slowly pushed down the food-rest of the recliner to create a normal chair. I was trying not to wake Becky, but the soft click, when the food-rest secured itself into the recliner, sounded like a metal wrench banging on a metal trash-can; way louder than it really was. I looked in her direction, but she remained asleep. My bare feet touched the cool laminated floor. My jeans and t-shirt were all wrinkled from the restless night. I found my white sport socks, jumbled up in a ball next to the recliner. After unfolding them, I slipped them on, and went on my way to find some coffee in the kitchen area.

The smell of sweet, fresh pastries, mixed with the bitter scent of coffee, welcomed me as I opened the door to the kitchen. The table was filled with pastries, sandwiches, cookies, fruit, and so forth. Many companies donated their left-over food to the hospice center, so there was always an overflow of goodies. The coffee pot was filled to the top. It seemed it was just recently made. Armed with a fresh cup of Joe, I returned to Becky's room. She was sitting straight up, wide awake.

"I was wondering where you went off to," she said.

"Just getting some coffee, sweetie," I answered as I placed it on the nightstand next to her bed. I leaned forward and gave her a gentle good-morning kiss.

"Morning babe," I said.

She smiled, touched my face, and pushed herself up to give me another kiss.

"I already ordered breakfast," she said. "The nurse just left."

A plate filled with eggs, a biscuit, grits (Becky's favorite), fruit and a cup of coffee was placed on top of the tray table. Becky was taking small bites of everything while she was staring outside. Suddenly, out of nowhere, she made a peculiar remark.

"Do you see those little baby birds outside?"

I stood up with my coffee in my hand.

Baby birds? I was thinking, *It's August, there are no baby birds...*

I walked over to the window, used my index finger and thumb to open up an area in the middle of the plastic slats. I did not see anything.

"No, sweetie. I do not see anything," I responded.

"Oh," she exclaimed, "they must be dead then. I have been seeing a lot of dead things lately," and she continued her breakfast as if it had been the most normal thing in the world to say.

Confused about what just had happened, I sat back down and sipped my coffee while Becky continued to eat her breakfast.

Some of the family arrived right after Becky was done eating. They would be staying with her the rest of the day so I could go home, get a shower, and hang with the boys for a little before we would come over and visit with Mama. Then I would take the boys somewhere to eat before I went back to stay the night at hospice.

The boys and I arrived later that afternoon. Connor and Dane were visiting with everyone that was there. Many people stopped by today since it was the weekend. We had placed some pictures from Connor and Dane in the room earlier that week. Suddenly Becky said,

"Connor, get that picture. There is something written on the back of it."

Her voice filled with panic as her finger pointed at the picture of him that was standing on the fireplace mantel.

"Get it! Get it!" she kept repeating.

Connor, with big confused eyes, raised one eyebrow and looked at me with an expression like *'what is going on here?'* I nodded at him, my lips without a sound instructed him to *'go-ahead.'* As he got to the picture, Becky was getting more and more filled with terror.

"Get it! Get it!" she said.

Once Connor got the picture to her, she placed it in her lap, flipped it over and started to push the little metal slides to open the back and expose the picture. When she lifted the black cardboard from the frame, the backside of the picture was just plain white, no writings. She pushed it to the side, and now more frantic she told Connor to get the next picture; the one with Dane on it.

"Honey," I said, "it's ok, let me get those pictures for you ok?" I tried to calm the situation.

I nodded to Connor for him to know I would take care of it.

Becky continued,

"There is something written on the back of those picture babe," she said with a determined look in her eyes.

Becky's mother tried to help and calm the situation also.

"Maybe we should write something on the back of it Becky, is that what you want to do?" she said.

Becky was not having any of it, she was not resting until she had seen all the pictures and made sure there were no writings on the back of any of them. After she checked all of them, as fast as this became an issue, it disappeared.

The drive home was different. I could see it in the eyes of both boys that they were really confused and shocked about what they had just witnessed. It was hard for everyone, but especially for them. They did not understand that this was not their mama, it was the disease, the medicine, the radiation or whatever was causing it.

"Mama was just really confused guys," I said.

"Yeah," Dane said, but Connor remained completely silent.

"Keep in mind that it is caused by all the medicine she is taking, the cancer, and the radiation of Mama's brain, okay?" I continued, trying to make sense of it all for them.

"I know," Connor replied.

Although they said they knew, the silence in the car was unavoidable. I needed to prepare them for what was coming. I needed to have that talk with them that no one wants to have. I needed to expose the painful horrific truth that everyone was trying to stick under the rug. I had to do this; it was my responsibility as their father. No one would help me with this one.

The drive home was about twenty minutes. At this time of the day, during the weekend, there were normally not many complications on the interstate unless an accident happened, then it could congest for hours. The boys ran upstairs to get their daily dose of X-box exposure. I stopped them halfway up the stairs.

"Hang on guys," I told them, "let's have a talk."

It is funny to realize how we are all creatures of habit. Automatically, both Connor and Dane sat down on the ottoman. Connor on the left, Dane on the right. They always faced the chair that Becky and I always sat in, because I would end up sitting there to talk to them. Today was no different. As we all took our seats, the uneasiness inside my body was eating straight through me. My stomach was in a knot and my hands were shaking. As I took my seat, even the soft comfort of the cushion, that would normally relieve stress, felt uncomfortable.

"Guys, things do not look really good right now," I said.

Connor's big eyes burned through my skin; Dane's silence beating me up.

"As you saw this afternoon, Mama is really confused at times. You need to know that at those moments, it is not Mama." My voice started to break apart, the shaking of my hands unstoppable.

"Mama has gone through a lot. All the medication, all the radiation, and all the other things," soft tears filled with pain started to pool in the corners of my eyes.

Slowly they escaped. With Connor and Dane in front of me, I usually tried to hide my pain, I did not want them to see my suffering, but I could no longer hold back.

"I think we need to be prepared for the worst boys," streams of raw pain were flowing down my cheeks.

Connor and Dane were both crying. Silently they sat in front of me, their eyes filled with tears and desperation. Their sniffles felt like sharp knives carving my soul.

"I do not think that Mama will come home from this place," I said, wiping my tears, breathing shallow, and uncontrollably shaking.

I placed my arms around them. We sat together holding each other, crying silently, tears falling onto the cold hardwood floor. Our souls were forever marked, engraved with a sharp blade of irreparable pain. Our lives would never be the same.

Becky was sound asleep when I arrived back at hospice. A family member stayed until I was back. She wanted to share a story with me that had happened earlier that day. Since Becky was asleep, we sat down in the sitting area across from her room. She explained that after the boys and I left, Becky made a remark about two men being in the room. Since there were no men in Becky's room, the family member decided to dig a little deeper and asked some questions about the two men that Becky was seeing. Becky explained that there were two men standing in the room facing her. They were there to make sure that she was okay. Becky explained that she knew the two men. Becky suddenly exclaimed,

"It is Larry and Danny!".

"Larry and Danny?" the family member asked Becky confused.

"Yeah," Becky responded, "They are here to tell me that everything is going to be okay,".

"Becky saw Larry and Danny!" the family member explained to me.

Larry and Danny were brothers. Danny was married to Becky's step-sister, and Larry was his brother. Larry was also our neighbor. Larry was also a fellow firefighter at the same fire department I was.

Ten years before, Danny, Larry, Larry's daughter and her fiancé were in a small plane crash, right before Christmas. All four of them did not survive that crash, it was a horribly devastating event. Now, according to this afternoon's appearance, both Larry and Danny had been there in Becky's room.

I chose to believe that they were there to help her, to guide her, to comfort her in the days to come.

That night was remarkably calm. Becky seemed to be asleep almost all night. Me on the other hand, could not stop watching her. It is weird that, when she was finally resting well, I wanted to watch her and make sure she was ok. I kept peeking over to her, to see if she was breathing, holding my breath to be quiet so I could hear her. The morning sun arrived too early, but I would always get up the moment the first rays of sunlight touched my face.

I found myself once again standing in the kitchen at the hospice-house, welcomed by the same smell of pastries and coffee. 'Just coffee' I was thinking, as I poured that black goodness into a mug. I blew onto the hot surface, sipping it gently.

"Ahh," escaped from my lips.

While walking through the hallway back to Becky's room, I noticed the beautiful garden that was placed in the middle of the building. I stepped outside through the door right next to the nurse's station. The cool summer morning breeze touched my face. I closed my eyes, lifted my head towards the sky and just breathed. Slowly in, slowly out, over and over again. I stood there like a frozen statue, holding my coffee cup, absorbing mother nature's scent, energy, and calmness. A hint of lavender was carried on top of the soft delicate breeze. I knew and understood, right there and then, why this was called the 'Healing Garden'.

When I walked back into Becky's room, she was still asleep. I opened the backdoor to the patio and sat down outside to enjoy the calm winds of that morning. I left the patio door open so I would be able to hear Becky. Around 9 am one of Becky's sisters came over to greet me outside. I welcomed her with a warm smile as she sat down in the other chair.

"How's Becky?" she asked.

"She slept all night," I responded, "and it seems she is still just snoozing away".

We talked for a little about nothing. When I emptied out my coffee-mug, it was time for me to go home and spend some time with Connor and Dane.

We said goodbye. I told her that I would be back later that afternoon with the boys. She smiled as I left the patio. Becky was still sleeping. Softly I placed a kiss on her cheek and whispered,

"I love you babe. I will be back later".

She did not respond. My fingers stroked her head as I placed one more kiss before leaving. When my lips touched her soft fragile skin, I closed my eyes and smelled her everlasting addictive scent. I just stood there with my eyes closed, my face against hers, my lips on her cheek, breathing in deep, exhaling slowly. Absorbing this loving moment. I did not want to go. I wanted to lay down next to her, hold her in my arms and just snuggle. Like we used to do every night before going to sleep.

The boys and I got there a little after 2pm. Although no one else would know or recognize it, I noticed some hesitation in them. The episode yesterday with the pictures had scared them a little. Today, Becky was doing great. She was very alert all day and stoked when the boys came in. They snuggled and kissed, and the boys crawled into her bed. Then Becky asked me if I could take some pictures of the three of them.

"Of course, sweetie," I said and pulled my phone from my pocket.

With both boys there, one on each side of her, she raised her arms up in the air and yelled,

"Cheese!!"

"You got it, you got it?" she asked.

"Let me check." I pulled up the picture and it looked great. I showed it to Becky.

"That's a good picture!" she said as she smiled.

The whole afternoon was fantastic. Time flew by. The boys had a great time and Becky seemed to have found some new energy. The nurse came in and asked Becky what she wanted to eat. I looked at my watch and noticed it was just a little past 4 PM. Since we were all doing great, I texted Lisa that we would stay a little longer.

'No worries,' she responded. *'Just let me know when you are on your way.'*

Becky was going over the food items that she could order, her finger flowing over the menu.

"What is chicken a la king?" she asked.

The nurse explained that it was rice with chicken, some vegetables and a special sauce.

"I will have that please," Becky said as she smiled.

Within fifteen minutes her dinner was served. A big bowl of chicken a la king, as ordered, served with some dinner rolls. When Becky started to eat, I decided it was time to take the boys home.

"I don't want to make it too late guys, since tomorrow is a school day," I reminded them.

"I know," Connor responded with a sad face.

"Let's get home and you guys can have dinner with Lisa ok?" I told them.

That for sure put a smile on their little faces since Lisa would probably take them to the local ice cream store afterwards.

Becky was hugged by the boys at the same time, from both sides. Many kisses were exchanged. Becky had wrapped her arms around them and squeezed them tight. She lit up the room with her big beautiful smile.

"Love you to pieces", she yelled as we left the room.

"Love you Mama," Connor and Dane responded as we walked out.

When I returned to Mercy Hospice later that evening, I parked my truck at the far south end of the parking lot. On these beautiful days, when the sun was still out and the temperature was comfortable in the mid to lower 80s, we kept the patio door of Becky's room open. Every room at this facility was facing the outside and had access to the yard surrounding the building. Each room had its own sitting area with a small table and a couple of chairs.

During dinner, Becky had eaten two bowls of the chicken a la king.

"That stuff is great honey," she said. "You should try some too."

"I will try some later, sugar," I said with a big smile.

The nurses were so nice and had already made my 'bed'. All I had to do was to crawl in, which I did. It was only eight PM, but I would just lay there, watch something on TV that I could watch without sound and eventually fall asleep. Becky's breathing was calm and deep. She had a great day today. I pulled up the blanket over my shoulders as I flipped on my phone, trying to find the picture I took earlier. There it was, both boys happy, Becky smiling. I had taken four pictures of them.

Then I noticed something I did not see before. I just thought she was just stretching her arms out wide to the air because of joy, but her hands caught my attention. Her hands made a symbol. A symbol that many know, but I was not expecting it to see here. With both her hands, the pinky and ring finger were together on one side, the index and middle finger together on the other side, creating a 'V' in the middle. *'Live-Long-and-Prosper'*.

What is up with that sign? What was going on this afternoon?

Suddenly everything started to become clear.

And what about that Chicken a la King stuff?

I knew she never liked that. Was that meal what I thought it was?

Twenty-One

As usual, I obtained my mug of daily caffeine from the kitchen at Mercy Hospice. But when I walked out, an unexpected visitor surprised me during my early morning routine. I was startled by the appearance of Doctor Freeman. His always addictive smile, topped with the eyes of an eight-year-old boy that did something mischievous, would make you immediately smile back. He was the last person I was expecting to see here. As we shook hands, he told me that he normally never comes to hospices to visit with patients.

"Don't get me wrong," he said, "but I am here to see you."

"Okay?" I said, somewhat confused. We sat down in the seating area across from Becky's room.

"I don't think you understand that you are quite unique," he said.

"I have seen many men run away from their spouses for less stress. You have fought this battle side-by-side with Becky. You never gave up, you never gave in, you continued your own research and you always stood by her. That is amazing, for I have seen people leave the sick one behind."

"I can't believe that people would leave their spouses because they have cancer," I responded.

He cleared his throat. "Roy, you would be amazed at the things we see, but yes, I have seen it. Some people just can't handle it."

"I also want you to know," he continued, "that when Becky developed the leptomeningeal metastases, I knew the statistics. Four to six weeks, and there is not much we can do about that. The fact that you refused to accept that news, and did all that research to find that study, ultimately gave Becky many more months."

It made me feel grand to hear all this from him. It was good to know that someone noticed and had the courtesy to tell me. Like when Stephanie, my fellow ER nurse, left that card in my locker.

"I just did what I thought was right," I said, "I assumed everyone would do that."

"Just know that I admire your commitment and persistence to help Becky," he concluded.

I walked back with him to the front door. While we were strolling down the hallways, we continued to talk about different issues. I started to wonder why he decided to tell me all this now. Why did he break his own rule to come here? Why not just call me? Right before I shook his hand, I realized his motivation was based on the fact that he was aware that he might never see me again.

Becky was in hospice. He knew what was going to happen. He knew that there would be no reason for us to meet anymore after we left this place. He needed to tell me this in person, but he was, up until now, unable to do so. He wanted me to know how he felt about this. That's why he came over that day. Our hands connected as I started to realize all this. My left hand joined the shake and locked his hand between both my hands to ensure he understood that I knew.

"Thank you so much Brian," I said. "It means a lot to me that you came out here to tell me this."

That morning for sure had a different start with the surprise visit from Doctor Freeman. I did not see my efforts in taking care of my sweetheart as unique, I just did what I thought was right. It was nice to receive a compliment, especially since I did not have the feeling I'd done anything extraordinary.

After Doctor Freeman left, I got a refill on my coffee from the kitchen, walked back to Becky's room and sat down in the recliner to read one of the books about dealing with grieving children that was given to me by one of the hospice nurses.

Lisa was going to take the boys to school, so I was just going to wait for a family member to come over so I could go home and clean up. I was rocking the recliner back and forth, sipping on my coffee, and flipping the pages of a book. I tilted the coffee mug upside down to drain the last possible sip from it. Becky was still asleep.

Odd, she is normally awake by now.

A soft knock on the door was followed by a female voice.

"Good morning," announced the arrival of one of the nurses.

"We are here to refresh the sheets."

As she walked through the doorway, another nurse followed her in.

"Good," I replied, "I need a refill on my coffee anyway."

I leaped out of the recliner and, as I walked past the nurse, we both smiled. On my return I noticed that the door was still closed. I did not want to interrupt so I decided to sit down on the love seat that was placed against the wall, right next to the door to Becky's room.

My eyes were just glaring at the garden behind the windows in the center of the facility. My mind was empty, just staring at nothing. Every now and then I would bring the cup to my lips to take a sip of coffee. From the corner of my eye I noticed one of Becky's sisters walking down the hallway. She smiled as she was getting closer. When she sat down next to me, she placed her hand on my leg and asked,

"How are you doing?"

"I am ok," I responded. "Just a little tired."

"How was the night?"

"Actually, pretty good," I said. "Becky slept very well."

At that moment, Becky's door opened. Both nurses came out and one of them just kept going while the other one stopped right next to me. The look in her eyes revealed that something had happened. She sat down and told me something that I did not want to hear.

"What's happening?" I asked her.

I looked her straight in the eyes so she was unable to avoid eye-contact.

"I think Becky is asleep," she said with.

"She just did not wake up at all when we replaced the sheets," she continued.

"We tried to wake her up a couple of times, but she is just not responding".

I felt the hand from Becky's sister moving away from my leg. It moved up to cover her mouth. Her face revealed shock and tears welled up in the corners of her eyes. Her voice silenced by pain.

My breath stopped, just for a brief moment, but long enough for the nurse to notice. She placed her hand on mine. Her eyes filled with care, understanding, and concern. No need for words, just silence. I took a deep breath in, followed by a long slow breath out. We all knew this moment was going to come, it was inevitable. But when it did, it felt like razor blades scraping the inside of my soul. The three of us just sat there, in silence, numb.

I waited until more family members had arrived before I drove home. The twenty-minute drive felt longer than ever. It was silent and lonely. The house felt cold and empty as I stepped foot into our home where we had lived for thirteen years. I sat down in our chair where we had spent almost every night together watching TV, watching the boys, or socializing with friends and family. Our chair was no longer occupied by us, just me.

For whatever reason the cat decided to show up. She jumped right next to me, onto Becky's spot. While she continued to face me, staring at me with big eyes, she crawled against me, softly purring, and then she rested her head on top of my leg without ever losing eye contact. My hand reached over to her amber colored, soft fur, and as I petted her, I asked,

"You know it, right?"

It was as if she knew what was going on. She closed her eyes and just laid there with me.

My heart broke into a thousand pieces, delicate streams of pain started to flow down my cheeks, my breath shallow and shaky, my shoulders jerking in small movements. My hand was on my forehead, covering my eyes. I could no longer resist and broke down. Tears dripped on the leather cushion of the seat, nose running, and my body shaking.

The fact that Becky was 'asleep', did not change anything about our schedule. I continued to stay every night with her, and someone would be with Connor and Dane. Every morning someone would come to Mercy hospice so I could go home, shower, then pick up the boys from school. I would take them to see Mama right after school till about 5pm. Then I would take them home, and someone would come over to take care of them so I could go back to hospice. We were all aware that Becky would probably not wake up again. Everything the hospice nurse told me four days ago was happening.

I noticed that there was a CD-player in Becky's room. So, I decided to bring some of her favorite music; Jimmy Buffet, Kenny Chesney,

Bob Marley, Barenaked Ladies, and Van Morrison. All day long Becky's room was filled with her favorite tunes. Frequently, whomever would be there, we would softly sing along.

Labor-day, 2013.

The sun broke through the windows. The hospice nurses had just come by to turn you to your other side. Your breathing had worsened over the last couple days. More frequently we had to use little sponge-swabs to remove the collection of saliva from your mouth. The nurses now only positioned you on your side to prevent aspiration. God, your breathing sounded so difficult.

It was becoming more agonizing by the day.

As the sun rays cut undisturbed through the room, it illuminated your left shoulder that was left bare. I noticed your pale, exposed skin. Fragile, delicate, once so easily to tan now discolored and gray. The thin, feeble protective layer, almost translucent, displayed windy curly blueish vessels. Some tiny, others large and bulky. I could almost see through that layer and detect the battle between the cells. It is an uneven and unfair battle in which the good slowly fades. The warmth of these sun rays would always stroke your skin to your pleasure, now you seem unaffected by its presence.

I am here, holding your hand, kissing your dried, cracked lips, stroking the side of your face. My head is laying against yours. My eyes might see your broken body, but all I experience is your divine beauty and kindness. I love you so much.

Connor and Dane were out of school, so we decided to go a little earlier to see Mama. She had been asleep now for a week. Every day after school, the boys and I would just sit with Mama for several hours. Family members would always leave the room when I would bring the boys, just to give us some privacy. I always recognized that, and I appreciated that. I am also sure they needed a little break from everything. Today was just a little different since they were out of school. We decided to go see Mama around 1pm. As usual we sat with Becky, but the boys were more active than normal.

"The boys are just wild today," I told the family. "I am going to take them home."

"Ok," they responded.

"I will be back around 4:30 or so," I said. "Lisa will be at my house at 4."

It was about 2:45pm when we got home. For some reason I found myself in a lot of discomfort. I kept pacing up and down the living room. My heart rate was up, and an unexplainable nervousness was eating me up from the inside. From the moment we left hospice, that feeling creeped inside and had intensified ever since. All I could think of was that I had to go back to Becky. After struggling with this feeling for fifteen minutes, I picked up my phone and called Lisa. After two rings she answered.

"What's up," she said with a concerned voice.

"Lisa, this is Roy, I just got home with the boys, but I have the feeling I have to get back to Becky as soon as possible. Can you come earlier?"

"I wish I could," she said, "but I am her until four."

"I just know I have to get back," I reiterated.

"Call Matt. I think he is home..."

I called Matt, her husband. He was home and said he was not busy and would be at my house in ten minutes. While I was waiting for his arrival, I grabbed clean pajamas for Becky. The nurse had asked me earlier to bring some. I was standing in our bedroom when I saw Matt arriving through the windows. I grabbed the bags with clothes and walked into the living room where Connor and Dane were sitting on the ottoman, their eyes fixated on the TV, playing an X-box game.

"Gotta go guys," I told them, as I kissed them both.

"Where are you going, Papa?" Dane asked.

"Back to Mama, okay? I will be back tomorrow."

"Okay," they responded in sync.

Matt opened the front door as I started to walk off the stairs.

"I am sorry I had to call you man," I said, "but I have the feeling I have to go back ASAP."

"That's okay," he responded. "I was not doing anything at home anyway."

I gave him a big hug, yelled one more, "Bye boys" and left.

The drive back to Mercy hospice was a torture. I do not know if I was getting mental, but the feeling of uneasiness was getting worse by the minute. I was not sure if I was just freaking myself out, but regardless, I had to get back to Becky. As soon as I pulled up in the parking lot towards the back of the facility, I parked my truck as close as possible to Becky's room.

From where I parked the truck, I could see her room. One of Becky's sisters was standing outside on the patio. She was on her phone. While I grabbed both bags of clothing, my phone rang. I answered.

"Roy, you got to get here now...Becky is not doing well..." It was Becky's sister that was standing on the patio with the phone.

"I am here right now," I said, "I just parked."

"Okay," she said. Her voice now trembling, pushing away tears.

"Hurry..."

With my phone in one hand, two bags of clean clothing in the other, I walked over to the backdoor of the room. Becky's sister was standing motionless on the patio, staring at me, with her eyes filled with sadness and tears that were almost breaking through. Her hand was in front of her mouth, waving at me to hurry up.

The back-patio door was on a crack. A gentle push with my elbow caused it to swing wide open. Family members were sitting around Becky. I could see her from where I was standing, slowly breathing, almost gurgling. Slowly in, slowly out...a pause...too long of a pause...then breathing again. A family member looked at me, and with a voice filled with fear,

"She started breathing really bad after you left."

My focus narrow, my mission clear. I dropped both bags on the ground and walked over to my girl. I fell to my knees right next to her bed. I leaned over and placed my face close to hers, my hand on her cheek.

"I am here baby," I said softly,

"...I am here..." I gently stroked her beautiful face.

I crawled onto the bed and laid my body down next to hers as carefully as possible, like a feather landing quietly on the floor. Her once so beautiful young radiant skin was cracking from dehydration, small flakes falling from it by every touch. Her ever fast-growing locks of shining hair were replaced by baldness as a result of the constant radiation. The brutal attack on her brain with gamma-rays to suppress the multiplication of the uncontrolled cellular structure known as cancer.

Her breathing was agonizing, short bursts in, long pause, soft short release, with a rate that was too slow for comfort. I knew she was hurting inside. I knew her soul was screaming for freedom. With my eyes closed, I could see the amazing beautiful spark in her eyes that emitted her beauty from within, and although her magnificent soul was harbored in this broken, sick, close-to-death body, her sheer beauty manifested itself through her radiant presence. No words were needed, no sight required, for I saw her from within. I felt the pure sensation of her loving presence next to mine.

I moved my face closer and placed my forehead against hers. With my eyes closed, I communicated to her, through my mind. I knew we could both hear each other without the spoken word. I'd heard her loud screams from miles away when I was at home earlier. As I softly folded my hand around hers and moved her arm around my upper body I whispered once again, now barely noticeable,

"I am here baby, it's ok...I am here."

As these words blew past my lips, I could feel my soul reaching out to hers to communicate the message of unconditional love with committed and dedicated passion. I placed my body closer to hers, just like we used to do every evening right before we would rest our souls for the night. My lips touched hers. Although they were cracked and dried out, I knew that her soul inside was young and full of life, ready to take the next journey and enlighten the world after this one.

My thumb softly caressed her cheek. I could feel the coolness of her skin. It caused the weird realization that this was it. Her shattered, sick body was shutting down. The end was close, ready to move on from this place to the next. Her breathing became less frequent, shallower, longer pauses...

Our souls connected 14 years ago and, through the years together, they became vigorously intertwined. We were soulmates for life. Without hesitation our love grew stronger, day by day, minute by minute. This entangled connection resulted in her soul reaching out to mine. When I was home with the boys, she wanted to assure my return to her. She was ready to travel but she did not want to leave me without a kiss, a touch, a goodbye. As I lay next to her damaged body, I felt her cool skin, I knew her soul reached out as I moved closer.

"I love you babe, it's ok," I whispered softly.

"I will take care of the boys. It's ok, don't worry about us."

The sudden tears that fell from my eyes were as raindrops nurturing the strength of our connection.

"It's ok babe...it's ok..."

Her lungs slowly exhaled, I felt her breath touching my lips, she squeezed my body with a determined strong grip, then...she relaxed. Her arm that was filled with a sudden strength that pulled me closer a brief moment ago was getting heavier. I felt the increasing pressure on my side. My eyes were closed, but I saw her clearly. I could feel her soul detaching...she relaxed more...there was no breath in...I noticed a cold chill...

The ear deafening silence provided the rude realization...you were gone...

***

The room is empty, cold rows of empty hard pews positioned to the left and the right of me. My path straight through the middle. No sound, just painful silence. Just you and I, like when we started fifteen years ago. I am holding your hand, my eyes to the ground. Tears falling, slow-motion splattering on the stone tiles, one by one.

Your hand is cold, your eyes are closed, your body motionless inside this uncomfortable box. Lipstick has been applied to your lips, but not as you would do it. It was missing precision; it was missing perfection. Your skin color is not yours. It has been plastered on, delicately and with care, but I know it is not your tone. I know this is you. My heart beats painfully.

My hand in yours, holding on, one more time. Without letting go, I bring my left hand closer. With my thumb and index finger I gently slide off your wedding band from my pinky. You gave it to me not that long ago. It was falling off your finger and I remember your words,

"I will get it back soon, when I gain some more weight."

I am breathing shallow with uncontrollable shivers coming from the core of my being. My cheeks are drowning in tears, the pain is unbearable. I wipe them away, trying to protect your delicate skin from my painful tears. I transfer our circle of endless love to your ring finger, and with delicate accuracy, I place the wedding band back to where it belongs. Your finger is cold, unnatural, and unable to bend. While it slowly passes your knuckle, I whisper,

"I do ..."

Our time is short, we only have a moment alone together, family is coming soon. I stroke my hand over your short hairs on your scalp, all that is left after the radiation so rudely destroyed your beautiful locks of hair. A lump in my throat, I have to stay strong, our boys are coming...my soul screams...

My lips touch your forehead, I am swallowing my pain.

"Forever and always," falls from my lips.

****** AFTERWORD ******

Sweet Becky,

It has been seven years since you were summoned to go where we all will meet again. During these years a lot has happened; good things and bad things, but I prefer to look at the good. You taught me to stay positive, no matter how bad, stay positive. You have given us many 'signs' for us to see. We are blessed with your guidance and we look forward to the years to come with more of your navigation. I am particularly thankful for your continued quest to ensure my happiness and showing me the way to a path that I have to travel.

Many times, I wondered and asked God only one question: Why?

Then, on a rainy afternoon when I was staring out the windows of our home, I realized that my whole life was molded to arrive at the moment where our souls met. We connected and moved forward together as one. The realization came that He placed me on your path to allow me to take care of you while you were facing this unfair, dreadful, and horrific battle.

Although disastrous, I am blessed that I was granted the honor to walk by your side during these dark times, to hold your hand and guide you through the night. Our souls were undetachable from the moment we connected. We were beyond words and at a higher level of communication through love. During the final moments, when I was blessed one more time to hold you close, to kiss your gentle lips before you took your flight, was a privilege. A unique blessing only for me.

You have filled me with true love and compassion, straight from your soul into mine. You will never leave me; you will always be here with us.

***

Becky and I never talked about death, we never talked about burial or cremation, but I knew Becky did not want to be stuck in a wooden box in the ground. Becky was and is a free spirit that wants to roam free. Placing her ashes in the ocean where her soul could always soar, was the only right choice. Even the location was simple: by Grandma Freddy, Washerwoman Shoal, Atlantic Ocean, Marathon Key.

Family members are a blessing and a challenge at the same time. When Becky was sick, many family members supported and helped. Some were so hurt and scared that they were unable to see how destructive their behavior was. I have talked to many widowers and widows about this. Most of them had similar stories. It is a very common dilemma, but most importantly, as I indicated, these 'attacks' normally are not personal. They are born from uncontrollable fear, pain, anger, frustration, and stress.

Without friends my journey would have been impossible. We had many friends that helped with almost everything. They are not all named in 'our story' but they know who they are. More importantly, Becky and I know who you are. We are grateful for your help and you will be locked inside my heart forever.

Grieving starts with the initial diagnosis. It does not wait till the day your soulmate leaves. From that moment on, you start to grieve about the ruthless devastation that is coming at you so fast. Grieving never stops, grieving is forever. Time does not heal any wounds; it allows you to deal with wounds differently. It continues to hurt, less painful but it will persist to sting from time to time.

CPSIA information can be obtained
at www.ICGtesting.com
Printed in the USA
FSHW010644220520
70362FS

9 781087 883502